Treatment of Eye Motility Disorders

Edited by Ivana Mravicic and Melisa Ahmedbegović Pjano

Published in London, United Kingdom

Treatment of Eye Motility Disorders
http://dx.doi.org/10.5772/intechopen.111150
Edited by Ivana Mravicic and Melisa Ahmedbegović Pjano

Contributors
Aditya Goyal, Alena Kolomytskaya, Alma Biscevic, Anja Shumejko, Blanka Doko Mandić, Fahd Kamal Akhtar, Ivana Mravicic, Ivona Petrovska, Jelena Škunca Herman, Lana Knežević, Maja Malenica Ravlić, Melisa Ahmedbegović Pjano, Natasa Draca, Nina Ziga

First published in London, United Kingdom, 2024 by IntechOpen
IntechOpen is the global imprint of INTECHOPEN LIMITED, registered in England and Wales, registration number: 11086078, 167-169 Great Portland Street, London, W1W 5PF, United Kingdom

British Library Cataloguing-in-Publication Data
A catalogue record for this book is available from the British Library

Additional hard and PDF copies can be obtained from orders@intechopen.com

Treatment of Eye Motility Disorders
Edited by Ivana Mravicic and Melisa Ahmedbegović Pjano
p. cm.
Print ISBN 978-0-85466-308-8
Online ISBN 978-0-85466-307-1
eBook (PDF) ISBN 978-0-85466-309-5

For EU product safety concerns:
IN TECH d.o.o., Prolaz Marije Krucifikse Kozulić 3, 51000 Rijeka, Croatia,
info@intechopen.com or visit our website at intechopen.com.

Meet the editors

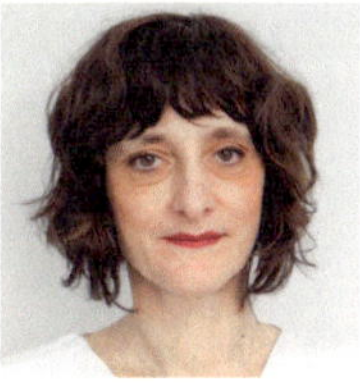

Associate Professor Ivana Mravicic, MD, graduated from the University of Zagreb Medical School, Croatia, where she completed her MSc and Ph.D. studies. She further developed her clinical and scientific skills with practical training in Munich, Zurich, Tubingen, and Hamburg. Professor Mravicic's field of interest is pediatric ophthalmology and strabismus. She has actively participated at more than 160 international conferences, published many scientific papers, and authored and co-authored several books and textbooks. Currently, she is the Head of the Paediatric Ophthalmology and Strabismus Department at the University Eye Clinic Svjetlost, Croatia. Dr. Mravicic also teaches ophthalmology at the University of Rijeka Medical School, Croatia.

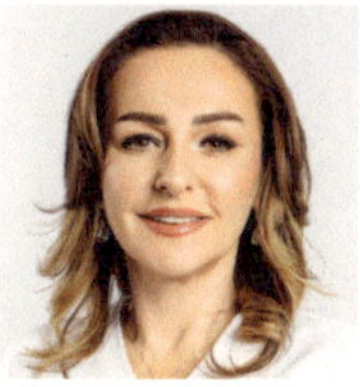

Melisa Ahmedbegović-Pjano graduated from the Faculty of Medicine in Sarajevo in 2001 and completed her ophthalmology specialization in 2005. From 2001 to 2011 she worked at the University Eye Clinic Sarajevo. She has been working in Eye Clinic Svjetlost, Croatia, since 2011. After completing postgraduate studies, she defended her master's thesis in 2010 and doctoral dissertation in 2017. She is engaged with the front segment of the eye and refractive surgery and has carried out around 15,000 laser vision correction surgeries to date. Her scientific interest is binocularity. Dr. Ahmedbegović-Pjano was elected to the position of assistant professor in 2023.

Contents

Preface

Our eyes are moved by six extraocular muscles that are innervated with the three cranial nerves. Both eyes are tuned to work together in every single moment and for the tiniest of targets. The proper, united functioning of both eyes enables the perception of depth, which is the last but not least perfection of our visual system. If disorders of eye motility are not properly treated in childhood during the developmental period, the visual system will not develop completely and, unfortunately, this malfunctioning cannot be improved later in life. When the motility of the eyes is not functioning in adult patients, every daily task becomes a problem. If eyes are not tuned properly, patients are unable to focus and can have asthenopia, headaches, and blurry vision. Another of the most prominent signs of an eye motility problem is double vision. Eye motility can be changed in some systemic diseases and therefore can be one of the first signs of a life-threatening disease. All of this points to the significance of proper and timely treatment of eye motility.

The introductory chapter explains the basic principles of the eye motility system and its disorders and gives a general guidelines of the treatment possibilities.

Chapter 2 describes tests and methods used to assess patients with eye motility disorders, with a special focus on the tests for binocularity and motility of the eye.

Chapter 3 focuses on different types of esodeviation, including types and subtypes as well as associated syndromes of esotropias.

Chapter 4 explains the etiology and epidemiology of exodeviation, including examination and treatment.

Chapter 5 discusses different types of conservative treatment for eye motility disorders.

Chapter 6 explains the treatment of paralytic eye motility problems, including the best surgical and nonsurgical choices.

I owe my greatest thanks to my boss, Professor Nikica Gabric, who has always supported me in my professional interest in ophthalmology. Professors Oliver Ehrt and Klaus Peter Boergen have played a great role in my passion for strabismus and pediatric ophthalmology.

I would also like to thank the authors for their excellent contributions.

I hope readers will find this book useful and informative and that it will help them in their everyday work.

Ivana Mravicic
Eye Clinic Svjetlost,
Zagreb, Croatia

Melisa Ahmedbegović Pjano
Eye Clinic Svjetlost,
Sarajevo, Bosnia and Herzegovina

Chapter 1

Introductory Chapter: Why, When, and How to Treat Eye Motility Disorders

Ivana Mravicic, Melisa Ahmedbegović Pjano and Natasa Draca

1. Introduction

Our everyday activities are more and more demanding, and we need not only perfect visual acuity but perfect stereoacuity as well to assess a clear image that is three-dimensional. Our eyes are positioned slightly apart from each other. This position enables our visual system to form two slightly different images of the same target on each eye. These images then travel into the visual part of the brain, where they are united in one single picture with the perception of depth. In order to create this image that is as close as possible to perfect, many conditions have to be fulfilled. A first condition for good visual acuity and depth perception is the formation of a clear image in each eye. The eye, with its refractive structures, has to be perfectly transparent with no refractive error in its structure. If there is a refractive error that is unrecognized and not corrected, the image of the eye will be blurred. In case one of the images is blurred, the brain cannot unite the distorted image from one eye with the image formed in the other good eye. In addition, if one eye is squinting, the visual target of the squinting eye will be different. Instead of two slightly different pictures that can be united in one perfect image, our brain will receive two different images from each eye, which will result in confusion or double vision. The capability of our visual system to perceive two slightly different images with each eye simultaneously is called binocularity [1]. Our brain then unites these two images in one single vision. This process is called fusion. However, even if we unite two slightly different images in one picture, there is still one more step to make this image three-dimensional. Uniting two images and forming a single one with depth is a function of the visual cortex and is called stereoacuity. It is already mentioned that our eyes have to be aligned to be able to perform one single vision of two slightly different pictures. For this precise alignment of the eyes, ocular muscles are responsible. There are six extraocular muscles that are responsible for eye movement. All of the muscles are innervated with cranial nerves. It is important to bear in mind that any process in cranium can affect cranial nerves, their nuclei, or structures adjacent to the nerves. Any of these can cause paresis or paralysis of the ocular muscle. Therefore, when treating patients with strabismus, we have to consider imaging and collaboration with neurologists, internal medicine specialists, or ENT specialists.

Eye motility problems can start in any age group. Sometimes, babies are born with squinting eyes. In such cases, early ophthalmological examination is obligatory in order to exclude anatomical reasons for squinting, such as congenital cataract or

IntechOpen

retinoblastoma, as well as some of the intrauterine infections. The main goal in the treatment of children with strabismus is to enable normal development of the eye. When children are born, they do not see well; their eyes, visual pathways, and visual cortex are not fully developed. In the cases when the eye cannot produce a good image of the target or cannot transfer it to the brain, the visual cortex of the affected eye will not develop normally. In children with squinting eyes, even if both of the eyes are healthy, the problem arises because the eyes are not aligned and the brain is receiving two different images, so to avoid double vision, the child's brain involuntary excludes one image and concentrates on the better one. With time, the squinting eye is less in use, and the lazy eye develops [2]. Since the plasticity of the brain and the ability to develop vision is limited to the early years, it is very important to enable normal visual input during the time when the visual system is developing [3]. When we have a small child with a squinting eye, our main goal is to enable proper development of both eyes. For that reason, surgery is not the only method of choice, and we have to prescribe glasses and patch the better eye. In the cases when squinting eye is not treated in childhood, it is possible to perform surgery later in life, but the result of the surgery will be only esthetic because the development of vision has already finished and cannot be improved anymore. The treatment of eye motility disorders is therefore obligatory in children. If an adult person has squinting eye that is not treated, or not successfully treated during childhood, treatment is possible, but it is only cosmetic. On the other hand, in the cases of newly developed eye motility disorders in older age, subjective symptoms of strabismus are usually much more dramatic because the brain of adults cannot adjust to the changes, so one of the most prominent signs is double vision. The line of diagnostics and treatment is different than in children. Excluding the cases when strabismus was present from an early age, every new eye motility problem in adult age has to be meticulously evaluated since the reason can be decompensated strabismus form earlier, but usually, it is some kind of vascular disease, compression, trauma, or, in some cases, disorder of hormonal or autoimmune system [4]. It is important to bear in mind that, in some cases, the reason behind strabismus can be life-threatening. After treatment of underlying disorder, if the eyes are not aligned, surgery is a method of choice. However, even in older age squinting can resolve spontaneously (e.g., recovery of the cranial nerve paresis), so it is recommended to wait for the surgery at least for 6 months. The treatment of eye motility disorders can be conservative or surgical.

2. Conservative treatment

2.1 Treatment by glasses

The first step in the treatment of a patient with strabismus of any age is the correction of refractive error. Refractive correction plays an important role in creating a sharp image on the retina, therefore promoting foveolar fixation. It also enables a proper balance between accommodation and convergence. Recommendations of prescription depend on the type of strabismus, age of the patient, and refractive error.

Patients with strabismus more often require the prescription of a full cycloplegic amount of refractive error, which can create difficulties in the acceptance of new glasses. The most common complaint is blurred vision at a distance in cases where a full amount of hypermetropia is prescribed because the patient is unable to relax accommodation. After several days, accommodation usually relaxes, and the patient, especially a young child, will accept new corrections. Another problem is that in children with strabismus, glasses have to be prescribed even when refractive error is physiological and visual acuity good, which might be difficult for both the parents and the child to accept. It is necessary to explain to parents why correction of the full amount of refractive error is needed. In the cases of accommodative (refractive) strabismus, the change in the deviating angle with and without glasses is dramatic [5].

However, many parents expect that strabismus will disappear completely after the glasses are worn for some time, so it has to be explained that glasses correct the position of the eyes and, by that, in children enable proper development of the visual system, but in cases when strabismus is not only refractive or accommodative, the eyes will squint even when the glasses are worn. However, in some patients with refractive accommodative strabismus, refractive correction can be the only needed therapy (followed by refractive surgery in adult age). Usually, it is only the first but necessary step in the treatment of strabismus, even if the surgery is eventually necessary. It has to be remembered that some studies have shown how full hypermetropic correction in a child's age can interfere with the process of emmetropization of the eye and should not be carried out routinely unless it is necessary in the cases of strabismus.

A special form of glasses is needed in the cases of accommodative esotropia with convergence excess. In these cases, bifocal lenses are used to reduce the angle for near vision and enable binocularity to develop. Bifocals in child's age should have the lower segment set high to the level of the pupilar axis. Instead of bifocal lenses, progressive lenses can be prescribed for older children.

Refractive correction can be used in some cases to blur the image in front of the fixating eye by over- or under-correction in order to change fixation preference and hide certain types of deviations like DVD.

In rare cases of insuperable diplopia, glasses or contact lenses can often be used to help patients ignore diplopia. The ability to ignore diplopia varies; in some cases, the reduction of vision can help the patient, but in others, it may require complete occlusion of the affected eye. If the reduction of vision is helpful, over- or under-correction in the glasses can be tried. In cases when complete occlusion is needed to ignore double vision, occlusive patches can be worn over the spectacles or painted lenses incorporated. Less obvious but effective can be neutral density filters. Occlusive correction can be worn in the form of contact lenses or occlusive intraocular lenses as well.

2.2 Treatment by prisms

Prism is a transparent, triangular refracting medium with a base and apex. A prism of one prism diopter (PD) power produces a displacement of 1 centimeter on an object that is situated 1 meter away. Light entering the prism will deviate toward its base, which will shift the image to the apex. On the other side, the prism has other unwanted optical effects, such as color dispersion and distortion of the image, which limits their clinical use. In patients with strabismus, prisms can be used for diagnostic or therapeutic purposes. Prescribing a prism can be a time-consuming and tiring task, but in the end, it can prove very helpful to the patient and worth all the time consumed. It is important to remember that before trying to help the patient with prism correction, all the other preconditions for good visual acuity and comfortable binocular vision have to be fulfilled (objective refractive error correction, exclusion of neurological or other medical conditions, assessment of binocularity). Criteria for the prescription of the prisms in the patient should be subjective problems (double vision, asthenopia, shift of binocular visual field); it is not recommended to prescribe prisms to the patient for cosmetic purposes. Cases that will most benefit are the ones with stress-dependent binocular problems (exo- or esophoria increasing during the day). The effect of the prisms has to be assessed in the office.

There are several types of prisms available.

Prisms can be incorporated into the glasses of the patient for continuous wearing, but care should be taken about the optical side effects of the prisms as well as the unsightly appearance and weight of such glasses. For these reasons, usually, not more than 5 PD in each eye is recommended.

Fresnel prisms are thin, narrow prisms that are arranged on a plastic sheet. In this kind of prism, the continuous surface of the prism is arranged as a series of steps. Fresnel foils are thin (1 mm) and flexible, and they can be cut into pieces that are applied to the back surface of the spectacles. Fresnel prisms are available in the power of 1PD-40 PD.

3. Surgical treatment

The last but not least option in the treatment of eye motility disorders is surgery. When the treatment of the underlying disease is completed, and conservative treatment is finished, surgery is the method of choice [6]. Although the reason for eye motility problems is sometimes situated in the visual areas of the brain or in cranial nerves, we can improve strabismus by performing surgery on extraocular muscles. Adjusting the muscle position and strength makes it possible to improve the position of the eyes and, in some cases, improve mobility. The most often performed surgeries are the weakening by recession (shifting backward tendon of the affected muscle) and strengthening with resection (shortening of the muscle-tendon). The amount of recession and resection is calculated based on the angle of deviation measured before surgery. Recession of 1 mm will correct 2 PD and a resection of 1 mm will correct 4 mm of squinting angle. In some specific cases, when the squinting angle is not the same for near and far distances, there is a possibility of performing some special type of surgery by splitting the muscle into two parts, which will change the lever arm of the operated muscle and correct only the near angle of deviation with much less effect at the far distance angle. To change action of the muscle, it is also possible to put an extra suture far behind the insertion to change the action of the operated muscle (posterior fixation or Faden surgery). In the cases of muscle palsy, it is possible to transpose adjacent well-functioning muscles or their parts next to the affected muscle and, by that, to some degree, improve the function of paretic or paralyzed muscle. There are several techniques available. In the cases when the muscle is too tight (dysthyroid orbitopathy, congenital fibrosis), a part of the affected muscle can be replaced with a prepared bovine pericard.

In conclusion, eye motility disorders can be congenital or acquired in any age group. They can be an isolated eye disease or connected with some systemic disorders or trauma. It is important to bear in mind the whole medical picture of the patient and have close cooperation with other medical specialties.

The treatment of high motility disorders is a demanding but interesting part of ophthalmology, with many conservative as well as surgical options for how to help our patients.

Author details

Ivana Mravicic[1]*, Melisa Ahmedbegović Pjano[2] and Natasa Draca[1]

1 Eye Clinic Svjetlost, Zagreb, Croatia

2 Eye Clinic Svjetlost, Sarajevo, Bosnia and Herzegovina

*Address all correspondence to: ivana.mravicic@svjetlost.hr

References

[1] Braddick OJ, Atkins J. Some recent findings on the development of human binocularity: A review. Behavioural Brain Research. 1983;**10**(1):141-150. DOI: 10.1016/0166-4328(83)90160-2

[2] Nye C. A child's vision. The Pediatric Clinics of North America. 2014;**61**(3):495-503. DOI: 10.1016/j.pcl.2014.03.001. Epub. 2014 Apr, 1

[3] Levi DM, Knill DC, Bavelier D. Stereopsis and amblyopia: A mini-review. Vision Research. 2015;**114**:17-30. DOI: 10.1016/j.visres.2015.01.002. Epub. 2015 Jan, 29

[4] Umapathi T, Koon SW, Mukkam RP, Chin LS, Beng TC, Helen T, et al. Insights into three dimensional structure of the oculomotor nuclear complex and fascicles. Journal of Neuro-Ophthalmology. 2000;**20**(2):138-144

[5] Reza, Akbari M, Heirani M, Kundart J, Christian L, Khorrami-Nejad M, Babak Masoomian B. Application of bifocal and progressive addition lenses in the management of accommodative esotropia: A comprehensive review of current practices. Survey of Ophthalmology. 2022;**67**(5):1506-1515. DOI: 10.1016/j.survophthal.2022.02.005. Epub. 2022 Feb, 17

[6] Lennerstrand G. Strabismus and eye muscle function. Acta Ophthalmologica Scandinavica. 2007;**85**(7):711-723

Chapter 2

Assessment of Binocular Vision

Aditya Goyal

Abstract

Assessment of binocular vision parameters comprise of quantified evaluations of the parameters. It is essential that these parameters are objective as far as possible and should resort to the laws and norms of ocular motility and space perception. This document on evaluation of binocular vision parameters begins with a brief discussion on anatomy, physiology of the binocular system and the laws governing it. These are followed by a detailed description of tests to assess accommodation, vergence and sensory status of the eyes. The tests have been explained and each of them have been described as a stepwise approach too to make the understanding easy to follow and perform. A brief classification of neuromuscular ocular disorders and non-strabismic binocular vision disorders is included at the end.

Keywords: binocular vision assessment, accommodation, vergence, sensory status tests, non strabismic binocular vision disorders

1. Introduction

In the world of computers and mobile devices, visual demands have increased multiple folds. Our eyes which were not meant to be used the way they are being used today need further and detailed evaluations. The mechanisms and the parameters of accommodation, vergences and binocularity require appropriate evaluation and interpretation of the data. Analysis of the findings and extrapolation of the data become the starting point to initiate vision therapies. These finally result in the reduction in symptoms and improvements in parameters ascertained initially.

2. Anatomy and physiology of extraocular muscles

Humans have 6 extraocular muscles in each eye. Four recti muscles move anteriorly from the orbit and get attached to sclera near cornea. Two obliques muscles arise from the medial aspect of the orbit, from there they continue obliquely and laterally, and insert into sclera posterior to the equator, on the temporal part of the globe. Contraction of recti muscles, pulls the globe backwards and nasally, whereas contraction of oblique muscles pulls the globe forward and nasally [1].

Recti muscles:

The recti are flat and narrow in appearance. They attach to the globe with thin tendons.

The four recti are:

1. Medial rectus

2. Lateral rectus

3. Superior rectus

4. Inferior rectus

The four recti, superior oblique, and levator palpebrae superioris originate at the orbital apex and are arranged in a circular fashion around the orbital opening and called the annulus of Zinn. Insertion of medial rectus is closest to the limbus, followed by inferior rectus, lateral rectus, and superior rectus.

Oblique muscles:

Superior oblique originates at the apex of the orbit. It runs anteriorly parallel to the upper part of the medial wall of the orbit. There it goes through trochlea and turns laterodorsally at an angle of 54 degrees with respect to the pretrochlear part of the muscle. This, then becomes tendinous towards the distal end, passes beneath superior rectus and merges laterally with the sclera.

Inferior oblique is the shortest of all the extraocular muscles. It arises in the anteroinferior angle of the orbit, from there it continues backward, upward, and laterally. It passes between the floor of orbit and inferior rectus and insert in the posterior and external aspect of sclera.

Centre of rotation:

The eyeball is presumed to perform rotary movements around a center of rotation, which is assumed to be within the globe. Presumably, the line connecting middle of lateral orbital margins goes through center of rotation of the two eyes.

As the eyeball is presumed to have a fixed center of rotation for practical purposes, the globe rotates in three directions going through the center of rotation.

1. Anteroposterior (Y axis)

2. Vertical (Z axis)

3. Horizontal (X axis)

The plane in which the vertical and horizontal movements take place is called Listing's plane, and is defined as the plane fixed in the orbit that passes through the center of rotation and the equator of the globe, with the eye in primary position.

Duction movements:

The rotation of one eye is called duction.

1. Rotation around Z axis: adduction/abduction

2. Rotation around X axis: elevation/depression

3. Rotation around Y axis: incycloduction/excycloduction

Movements around "Z" and "X" axes are called cardinal movements, and a combination of these cause oblique movements which are around "Y" axis.

Positions of the globe:

When a person is looking straight ahead with the body and head erect, it is called primary position.

Adduction, abduction, elevation, and depression are secondary movements and oblique positions are tertiary positions of the eye.

Actions of muscles:

1. Lateral rectus abducts and medial rectus adducts the eye from the primary position.

2. In primary position, superior rectus not only elevates but also rotates the eyeball causing incycloduction and adduction. Inferior rectus on the other hand, depresses the globe, excycloducts and has a slight adducting action.

3. Superior oblique causes incycloduction, depression and abduction whereas inferior oblique causes, excycloduction, elevation and abduction.

Versions:

These are binocular movements of the eyes in the same direction. These movements enlarge the field of view and help in bringing the object of interest on the fovea. Versions are fast movements and can be voluntary or involuntary.

Stimuli in the retinal periphery elicit saccadic eye movements, which are fast movements to place the object of regard on the fovea and keep it there. Pursuits track a moving object. The function of saccades is to correct the position error between target and fovea, whereas that of pursuit is to match eye velocity to target velocity.

Vergences:

These are binocular movements of the eyes in opposite directions. Vergence movements align the eyes to ensure and maintain binocular fixation and binocular vision. These are slow movements as compared to versions.

Convergence occurs when an object approaches the eyes and divergence occurs when it recedes. Vergence movements are made for fusion and are required for fusional vergences. Cyclovergences are compensatory adjustment movements to correct the relative position of eyes in the presence of vertical or cyclophorias.

Laws of ocular motility:

Contraction of extraocular muscles brings about movement of the eyeball. Muscles responsible for bringing about this movement are called *agonists*. Muscles that move the eyeball in the opposite direction to that of agonists are called *antagonists*. Medial rectus adducts the eyeball and lateral rectus abducts it. Hence medial rectus and laeral rectus are antagonists.

Two muscles that move the eyeball in the same direction are called *synergists*. Superior oblique and inferior rectus depress the eyeball, they are synergists for that, but for cyclorotation they are antagonists as superior oblique incycloducts and inferior rectus excycloducts the eyeball.

Considering binocular actions, two synergistic muscles moving both the eyes in the same direction are called *yoke muscles*. Right medial rectus and left lateral rectus cause levoversion of the two eyes. They are yoke muscles.

A pair of muscles in one eye can be yoked with a pair of muscles in the other eye. Elevators of one eye are yoked with the elevators of the other eye. Yoking also changes with the eye movements. The right medial rectus is yoked with the left lateral rectus for lateroversion, however, medial recti of both eyes are yoked for convergence.

Sherrington's law of reciprocal innervation:

Whenever an agonist receives an impulse to contract, an equivalent inhibitory impulse is sent to its antagonist to relax. This law is applicable to all the striated muscles of the body and not extraocular muscles alone.

Hering's law of equal innervation:

Whenever an impulse is sent to an extraocular muscle, corresponding muscles of each eye receive equal innervations to contract or relax. This is also called the law of motor correspondence. Unlike Sherrington's law, Hering's law applies only to extraocular muscles.

Isolated innervations to an extraocular muscle do not occur, nor can the muscles of one eye alone be innervated. Impulses for ocular movements are integrated and all ocular movements are associated.

3. Tests for binocular functions

Assessment of binocular functions involves examination of ocular motilities, presence of any kind of motility problems like inaccurate saccades or pursuits, speed deficits in motility etc. Binocular status must be assessed for alignment in all the cardinal directions of gaze [2–4].

3.1 Extraocular motilities

This test is done to check the ability to perform conjugate eye movements (i.e. both the eyes together).

A penlight is held directly in front of the patient's eyes at about 30 to 40 cm. This is the "primary position" of the eyes. Then, the light is moved in eight cardinal directions. (It will resemble a figure "H" bisected by a vertical line).

Patient is instructed to follow the light with his eyes, without moving the head. He or she is also instructed to report if the light appears double in any direction or if any pain or discomfort is experienced. Examiner should note the smoothness, accuracy & extent of movements.

If the ocular movements are full, smooth, and accurate, then it is recorded as "FROM" (full range of movements). Otherwise, record the problem in movements. For example: jerky, nystagmoid movement in a specific gaze. If diplopia is experienced, it must be recorded in the specific direction of gaze and should be followed by diplopia charting.

Procedure in steps:

1. Patient is instructed to follow the light in different directions with his eyes and report if he or she experiences double vision, pain, or discomfort.

2. Penlight is held in primary position and then moved in different directions of gaze.

3. Note the corneal reflex, smoothness, and accuracy of movements.

4. If everything appears normal, then record it as "FROM" (full range of ocular motility), otherwise note the deficits.

5. If the patient complains of diplopia, note the direction in which it was observed by the patient and perform diplopia charting.

Muscle imbalances can cause turning of the eye/s in, out, up, down, or tendencies to do so. Eso is a turning in, exo is a turning out, hyper is a turning up, and hypo is a turning down. A phoria is a *tendency* to turn, while a tropia is a *definite* turning of the eye. Therefore, esotropia is a definite turning in, while an exophoria is a tendency to turn out. Hypotropia is a definite turning down, while hyperphoria is a tendency to turn up.

Strabismus is a condition in which the eyes are not aligned appropriately. It is also referred to as a squint or crossed eyes and may lead to *Amblyopia*. Strabismus and Amblyopia are the most common causes of visual impairment in children. Different tests are used to assess and quantify latent and manifest squint. Most of these tests are objective and do not require patient's response.

3.2 Bruckner test

This test is usually performed in infants and preverbal children. It is to screen for binocularity by comparing the brightness of red reflex from the pupils of both the eyes.

A direct ophthalmoscope with a large spot of illumination is directed towards the patient's eyes from a distance that is sufficient to cover both the eyes (usually about 1 meter), with the patient looking at the spot. Examiner views the red reflexes in both the pupils through the peephole of the scope.

Brightness of reflexes from both the pupils is compared. Equally bright reflexes indicate binocular fixation. If they are not equally bright, the brighter one indicates a non-fixating eye. This difference in brightness may be due to strabismus, anisometropia, anisocoria etc.

If the reflex appears unequal, record the eye from which the reflex appears brighter.

Procedure in steps:

1. A large spot of light from a direct ophthalmoscope is directed towards the patient's eyes from approximately 1 meter.

2. The examiner views the reflex from the pupils through the peephole of the scope.

3. Reflexes are compared for brightness.

4. Observation is recorded as reflex appearing equal or unequal. If it is unequal, then record the eye which shows a brighter reflex.

3.3 Hirschberg test

This test is performed to determine the approximate position of visual axes at near, thus identifying strabismus and quantifying it approximately.

Penlight is directed towards the patient's eye from about 50 cm, with the patient viewing it directly. The location of corneal reflex in both the eyes are viewed. If they appear centered, then the patient does not have strabismus, otherwise he or she has strabismus.

The size of strabismus can be estimated by measuring the distance between the expected and the deviated positions. One millimeter of deviation is equal to 22 prisms.

Strabismus can be approximated quantified in the following way:

1. If the reflex appears at the edge of the pupil, then the deviation is approximately 15 degrees.

2. If it is centered between the edge of the pupil and the limbus, then the deviation is about 30 degrees.

3. If the reflex is at the limbus, then the deviation is quantified to be approximately 45 degrees.

The relationship between the position of the corneal reflex and the type of deviation is as follows

1. If the position of the reflex is nasal to the centre of the pupil in the deviating eye, then there is exotropia.

2. If the position of the reflex is temporal to the centre of the pupil in the deviating eye, then there is esotropia.

3. If it is above the centre of the pupil, then it is hypotropia relative to the fixating eye.

4. If it is below the centre of the pupil, then there is hypertropia relative to the fixating eye.

Procedure in steps:

1. Light from a penlight is shown from about 50 cm with the patient viewing it directly.

2. Examiner looks for the corneal reflex.

3. Position of the corneal reflex is noticed, and if the reflex is not centered, then the strabismus is approximately quantified depending on the location of its position in the deviated eye.

4. Recording is accordingly documented.

The quantification can be measured by placing prisms in front of the deviating eye.

3.4 Krimsky test

This is an extension of Hirschberg test to quantify the amount of strabismus. On noticing the deviation, a prism with its apex towards the deviation is placed in front of the deviating eye. For example, in case of exotropia, a prism is placed with its base in, in front of the deviating eye.

The amount of prism is gradually increased until the corneal reflex is in the same relative position in the deviating eye as it is in the fixating eye.

In case of scarred cornea or very poor visual acuity in the deviating eye, an alternate procedure called modified Krimsky is used. The procedure is same as Krimsky, except that the prism is placed in front of the fixating eye.

To avoid parallax error, it is ideal for the examiner to view the corneal reflex with one eye closed.

Procedure in steps:

1. If a deviation is noticed on Hirschberg test, a prism is placed in front of the deviating eye, with its apex towards the direction of deviation.

2. The amount of prism is increased until the reflexes in both the eyes appear centered. This is the amount of strabismus that the patient has.

To identify and differentiate between phoria and tropia, cover – uncover test and alternate cover test is used. These tests help in differentiation as well as quantification of the squint.

3.5 Cover test

This test is performed to evaluate the presence of phoria or tropia. The cover test assesses the presence or absence of motor fusion. Motor fusion is responsible for bringing about alignment of the eyes.

This test is performed both for distance and near. When it is done at near, accommodation and accommodative convergence comes into play. The test is performed with the patient wearing the best correction for refractive error. For distance, the target is one line larger than the best visual acuity in the poorer eye. For example, if the patient has 20/20 in the right eye and 20/30 in the left eye, then, 20/40 line is isolated to perform the test. Target for near is an accommodative target held at 40 cm. For this too the line larger than the best visual acuity in the poorer eye is isolated for the test.

An occluder is held by the examiner to cover one of the eyes. The examiner is positioned in such a way that the patient's view of the target is not obstructed, and the examiner is able to view any movements of the eyes.

3.6 Cover: Uncover test

This test, as mentioned before, differentiates between phoria and tropia. It also helps in differentiating between an alternating or unilateral tropia.

As the first step, fixating eye is covered by the occluder, with the patient fixating the target at distance. The occluder is held in front of the eye for a few seconds before the eye is uncovered. Examiner should look for any movement of the uncovered eye. After a few seconds of covering, the occluder is removed and the eye which has been uncovered is observed as soon as the cover is removed. Then, the other eye is covered, and similar observations are made.

If the patient has tropia, then the uncovered eye will take up fixation showing the presence of tropia. If there is no movement seen, then there may be phoria or the patient may be orthophoric.

When the cover is removed from the fixating eye, and the just uncovered eye shows a movement, it is indicative of the presence of phoria. This is seen because when both the eyes were uncovered, the patient was using fusional vergences to maintain alignment. However, on covering one of the eyes, the fusion was broken and the phoria gets uncovered.

If there is no movement seen on covering or uncovering either of the eyes, then the patient is orthophoric.

Cover – uncover test is also used to differentiate between alternating and unilateral tropia.

1. If the right eye is covered and the left eye takes up fixation and returns to the deviated position on uncovering right eye, then the patient has tropia in the left eye.

2. If, on uncovering the right eye, the left eye retains fixation, and the right eye takes up deviated position, then the patient has alternating tropia.

The same procedure is repeated for a near target at 40 cm. This provides information about phoria or tropia with the accommodation and accommodative convergence mechanisms acting. If a patient is orthophoric for distance but has deviation for near, then it is because of the accommodation/convergence mechanism.

3.7 Alternating cover test

The settings are same as in the cover test. Patient is required to fixate the line on the distance chart. Examiner covers the right eye with the occluder and after a few seconds quickly shifts it to the left eye. This procedure of alternately covering and uncovering is carried out several times, making sure that either of the eyes is kept covered to disrupt fusion.

After the direction of the deviation has been determined, magnitude of deviation can be measured by placing prism bar in front of either eye. After interposing the prism bar, the amount of prism is increased gradually until no movement of the eye on alternate cover test is seen. This is also referred to as prism bar cover test (PBCT). Alternate cover test is similarly performed for near, with the patient fixating a near line larger than the best visual acuity in the poorer eye.

3.7.1 Relationship between eye movement and the direction of deviation in the deviating eye when the fixating eye is covered

See **Table 1**.

Prisms required for neutralizing the movement:

1. For exo deviation, prism with its base in is used.

2. For eso deviation, prism with its base out is used.

	Direction of eye movement	Direction of deviation
1	In	Exo
2	Out	Eso
3	Up	Hypo
4	Down	Hyper

Table 1.
Interpretation of type of tropia based on the direction of eye movement.

3. For hypo deviation, prism with its base up is used.

4. For hyper deviation, prism with its base down is used.

Procedure in steps: (cover – uncover test)

1. For cover – uncover test, the fixating eye is covered with an occluder, while the patient is fixating an isolated line in the distance Snellen's chart.

2. The examiner looks for movement of the eye which is not covered.

3. If the eye which is not covered moves, then the patient has a tropia.

4. If it does not move, then it could be a phoria or the patient may be orthophoric.

5. The covered eye is uncovered, and the examiner looks for movement of the uncovered eye immediately on uncovering it.

6. If a movement is seen, then the patient has phoria.

7. If no movement was perceived, then the patient is orthophoric.

8. If tropia was noticed, and on removal of cover, the eye goes back to its deviated position, then the patient has unilateral tropia.

9. If the uncovered eye retains fixation, and the phenomenon repeats on covering and uncovering the fellow eye, then the patient is said to have alternating tropia.

10. Test is repeated in the same way for a near target

Procedure in steps: (alternating cover test)

1. This test is to determine the magnitude of deviation seen in cover – uncover test on incorporation of prisms in front of the deviating eye.

2. Both the eyes are covered alternately, without leaving either of them uncovered to avoid fusion.

3. A prism bar in placed over the deviating eye, and alternate cover test is performed to see the movement of the eye.

4. The amount of prisms is gradually increased, until no movement of either eye is perceived on alternate cover test.

5. This is the amount of deviation of tropia or phoria.

6. The test is repeated for a near target and the deviation for near assessed.

4. Tests to evaluate sensory status

To avoid diplopia in strabismus or aniseikonia in clinically significant anisometropia, several sensory adaptations manifest. They are [2, 5]:

1. Suppresion

2. Anomalous retinal correspondence

3. Amblyopia

In suppression, the patient may have normal visual acuity in both the eyes, but one of the eyes (usually the deviated eye in strabismus) is suppressed to avoid diplopia. These patients do not have binocular vision though they may have normal monocular visual acuities.

For a complete binocular visual status, it is important to attain the three grades of binocular vision.

1. Simultaneous macular perception

2. Fusion

3. Stereopsis

When an object is imaged simultaneously on maculae of both the eyes, then a person is said to have simultaneous macular perception. In a patient who has strabismus, due to the deviation, simultaneous macular perception does not take place and the image falls on an extrafoveal point. Sometimes, in strabismus, an anomalous correspondence takes place between the macula of one eye and an extrafoveal point of the other eye. This, as mentioned before, is a sensory adaptation.

Fusion is the ability of the brain to form a single image by coordinating the movements of the two eyes so that the visual images fall on corresponding areas of the retinas of the two eyes. This can be sensory or supported by motor activity.

To assess fusion ability at different distances, a Worth 4 dot test is used. This test also shows if the patient is suppressing either of the eyes or has diplopia.

4.1 Worth four dot test

This test is performed at different distances. The target comprises of four colored dots. They are arranged in a diamond shape. Usually, red dot is at the top, white at the bottom and two green dots on the sides.

The patient wears his correction and red – green glasses are worn over it, with red in front of the right eye and green in front of the left eye. It is important to check the cancelation of the target colors with the filters. The patient is required to tell how many dots he sees, their colors and respective positions.

The test is similarly performed for different distances using a handheld Worth 4 dot flashlight.

Responses that may be given and their interpretation:

1. If the patient reports that he sees four dots, then he has flat fusion.

2. If the patient sees only two red dots vertically, then he is suppressing his left eye.

3. If the patient reports seeing three green dots alone, then he is suppressing his right eye.

4. If he or she reports seeing five dots, then ask the patient where the green dots (seen by the left eye) are located with respect to the position of the red dots (seen by the right eye). Based on the response, relationship of the visual axes can be determined.

5. If the red dots are to the right of green dots, then the patient has eso (uncrossed) deviation.

6. If the red dots are to the left of green dots, then the patient has exo (crossed) deviation.

7. If the red dots are above the green dots, then there is left hyper deviation.

8. If the red dots are below the green dots, then there is a right hyper deviation.

9. The distance at which the patient reports suppression, provides an idea about the size of the suppression scotoma. For example, if the reported suppression is at a very close distance from the patient, then the size of suppression scotoma is big as compared to a small suppression scotoma if it is reported at a far distance.

Procedure in steps:

1. The patient wears red – green glasses over the habitual correction, with red in front of right eye and green in front of left eye.

2. He or she is requested to look at Worth 4 dot test, projected at different distances.

3. Patient's response about the number and relative position of different dots is elicited.

4. Based on the response, diagnosis is ascertained.

After the patient's ability to fuse has been ascertained, it is important to measure the final grade of binocular vision – stereopsis. This is done to measure the patient's depth perception through his or her ability to fuse stereoscopic targets.

There are different tests used to measure stereopsis. Most of them require the patient to wear red – green or Polaroid glasses. There are some tests like Lang stereo test, which do not require use of either of these glasses. These tests are primarily used for very young children.

Usually employed stereopsis tests are:

1. Randot test

2. Titmus fly test

3. Bernell stereo test

4. TNO test

In all these tests, varying degrees of depth is perceived on wearing red – green or Polaroid glasses. The patient reports the same and it is recorded in seconds of arc. The depth in the targets is created by changing the disparity between them.

4.2 Stereopsis

The patient wears either Polaroid or red – green glasses over the near correction. A stereo test booklet is presented to the patient at 40 cm and his or her attention directed towards the smallest set of targets. The patient is asked to identify which of the circles in the set of circles appears to be floating above the plane of the booklet.

If stereopsis is appreciated, then he or she is instructed to go to the next set of targets. Continue this procedure until the patient reports two consecutive wrong replies.

Record the stereopsis in seconds of arc (mentioned in the instruction booklet supplied with the test) for the last correct response obtained from the patient before two consecutive incorrect responses.

Procedure in steps:

1. The patient wears red – green or Polaroid glasses over the near correction.

2. Stereo test booklet is presented at a distance of 40 cm.

3. The patient is asked to identify the circle which appears above the plane of booklet, in a set of circles shown to him or her.

4. Test is carried on until the patient gives two consecutive incorrect responses.

5. Amount of perceived stereopsis is recorded in seconds of arc.

When the patient has a mild reduction in monocular visual acuity and slightly reduced stereopsis, then, a very small central scotoma is suspected. This central suppression could be secondary to a small angle strabismus.

To confirm or rule out the presence of a small central scotoma or a small central suppression, 4 prism base out test is performed.

4.3 Four prism diopter base out test

The patient wears his best correction for distance. He or she is required to fixate at an isolated letter, one line above the best visual acuity in the poorer eye, on the distance chart. The patient is instructed to fixate on the target and try to keep it single all the time. The examiner holds a 4 prism with its base out in front of the better eye. The fellow eye is watched carefully for any movement.

Normal response is an outward comitant movement of the fellow eye, followed by an inward refixation movement. The prism should be held in front of the eye for refixation movement to take place.

As the next step, prism is held in front of the fellow eye (poorer visual acuity). Normal response is an outward movement of the fellow eye, followed by an inward refixation movement. The prism should be held in front of the eye for refixation movement to take place.

Expected results:

1. Normal result indicating no suppression of either eye: When the prism is placed in front of the right eye, the left eye moves out (Hering's law). The patient experiences diplopia, and to avoid that, an inner refixation movement takes place. Similar phenomenon is seen when the prism is placed in front of the left eye.

2. Abnormal result indicating suppression of the poorer eye: When the prism is placed in front of the better eye, the fellow eye moves outwards in consistence with Hering's law. However, as the fellow eye has a small suppression scotoma, the patient does not experience diplopia and hence no refixation movement is seen. When the prism is shifted to the suppressing eye, it does not experience shift in retinal image, and hence no movement of either eye is elicited.

Procedure in steps:

1. The patient wears his or her best correction for distance.

2. He or she fixates an isolated letter, which is from one acuity line better than the acuity in the poorer eye.

3. A 4 prism with its base outward is placed in front of the better eye and the movement of the fellow eye watched.

4. Then the prism is shifted to the other eye, and again the movement of the fellow eye is looked for.

5. In case there is no suppression, then fellow eyes in both the cases show a movement outward, consistent with Hering's law and then, an inward refixation movement is seen.

6. If the prism is placed in front of the suppressed eye, then no movement of either eye is seen.

7. When the prism is placed in front of the better eye (the other eye suppressing), then, an outward movement of suppressing eye is elicited (Hering's law), but no inward refixation movement is seen as the patient does not experience diplopia.

Once different grades of binocular vision have been evaluated, tests to ascertain accommodative and vergence system are performed. Clear, comfortable binocular vision depends upon several skills. One should be able to align the eyes and maintain it for a certain period. The patient must have sufficient amplitude of accommodation and must possess the ability to sustain it appropriately and efficiently. The accommodation and vergence mechanism must interact properly.

On ascertaining these values, the examiner decides if the patient's problems can be corrected with the spectacle or if he or she requires binocular vision training. Patient's spectacle prescription influences the accommodation and vergence systems and vice versa. Based on the findings, the examiner must decide if the correction requires to be revamped or not.

5. Measurement of latent deviation

Latent deviation or phoria is seen when fusion is disrupted. Both the eyes maintain alignment with the help of motor fusion. Accommodation convergence mechanism plays a big role in maintenance of this alignment. Sometimes, there is a great stress on this system, which results in aesthenopic symptoms. By proper measurement of phorias and vergences, one can diagnose the cause for aesthenopia and then treat it with optical devices or vision training. There are several methods to measure phorias. A few of them are [2, 3]:

1. Maddox rod method

2. Modified Thorington method

3. Von Graefe technique

Phoria is measured both for distance and near. It is also evaluated laterally and vertically. Finally fusional vergences are measured to ascertain the entire vergence mechanism.

5.1 Maddox rod method

This method of phoria measurement is used for lateral (horizontal) and vertical phoria for both distance and near.

The patient wears his or her correction, and a red or white Maddox rod is introduced in the trial frame in front of his right eye. A spot of light is switched on at six meters and the patient is instructed to look at it.

Maddox rod should be aligned in the following way:

a. For measuring lateral phoria, grooves of Maddox rod should be aligned horizontally, so that the streak appears vertical.

b. For measuring vertical phoria, grooves of Maddox rod should be aligned vertically, so that the streak appears horizontal.

Prisms should be introduced in front of the right eye in the following way:

a. For measuring lateral phoria, sufficient base in prism is introduced in front of the right eye. (They may be handheld or prism bar). This is done to move the streak of light to the right of the spot of light.

b. For measuring vertical phoria, sufficient prisms with base up orientation are introduced in front of the right eye. (They may be handheld or prism bar). This is done to move the streak of light below the spot of light.

The patient is instructed to look at the spot of light and be aware of a streak and a spot.

For lateral phoria measurement, reduce the amount of base in prisms until the patient reports that the streak of light is bisecting the spot. Record the prism value and the base orientation.

For vertical phoria measurement, reduce the amount of base up prisms until the patient reports that the streak of light is bisecting the spot. Record the prism value and the base orientation.

Similarly, phoria is measured for near using a penlight held at 40 cm by the examiner.

Procedure in steps:

1. The patient wears the correction and the Maddox rod (oriented horizontally for horizontal phoria and vertically for vertical phoria measurements) is placed in front of the right eye.

2. Sufficient prisms with base in orientation (for lateral phoria) and base up orientation (for vertical phoria) are placed in front of the right eye.

3. A spot of light is switched on at six meters and the patient is asked to look at it.

4. In case of lateral phoria measurement, the patient sees a streak of light with the right eye, which is to the right of the spot (displacement is due to the prisms incorporated) and with the left eye he sees a spot of light.

5. For vertical phoria measurement, with the right eye, the patient sees a streak of light, which is below the spot (displacement is due to the prisms incorporated) and with the left eye he sees a spot of light.

6. Prisms are reduced by the examiner until the patient reports that the streak bisects the spot of light.

7. The test is similarly carried out for near, with the patient looking at the penlight held by the examiner at 40 cm.

8. Amount of prisms and their base orientations are recorded as the measurement of phoria.

5.2 Modified thorington method

This test is performed to check lateral and vertical phoria for near. Thorington card is used to perform this test. This card is held 40 cm from the patient. The separation of numbers is such that at 40 cm, the spacing between any two numbers is one prism. There is a hole in the center of the card, through which penlight provides a source of light.

The patient wears his correction, over which a Maddox rod is placed in the trial frame in front of the right eye. For measuring lateral phoria, Maddox rod is oriented horizontally, and the streak appears vertical to the patient.

The Thorington card is held 40 cm from the patient with penlight at the center of the card. He is instructed to look at the light and tell the examiner if the streak is to the right or to the left of the light. If the streak is to the right of the light, then patient has esophoria, and if it is to the left, then it suggests exophoria. The size of the phoria is determined by asking the patient to tell the number through which streak passes.

For vertical phoria, the same procedure as in the measurement of horizontal phoria is used with the Maddox rod oriented vertically and a Thorington card with vertical rows of numbers is used. In this case if the streak passes through the light, it is orthophoria. If it is above the light, then the patient has left hyperphoria and if it is below the light, then it is right hyperphoria.

Size and the direction of phoria is recorded accordingly.

Procedure in steps:

1. The patient wears his or her usual near correction with Maddox rod in front of the right eye.

2. Maddox rod is oriented horizontally for lateral phoria and vertically for vertical phoria measurements.

3. Thorington card is presented to the patient at 40 cm distance, with penlight shown through the centre of the card.

4. The patient reports the number which is bisected by the streak and also the location of streak relative to the light.

5. Same method is used to measure vertical phoria except that vertically oriented Thorington card is used, and Maddox rod is placed with its grooves oriented vertically.

6. Phoria for both horizontal and vertical orientation is recorded.

6. Tests for vergence

When an object is brought closer, both the eyes converge to look at it. There is a synkinetic triad, wherein when an object is brought closer, accommodation, convergence and pupil constriction takes place simultaneously [2, 3].

If the near point of convergence recedes, it leads to aesthenopic symptoms. NPC (near point of convergence) is a measure of convergence amplitude – the maximum ability to converge while maintaining sensory fusion.

1. NPC Break (Objective) – The point where the patient can no longer maintain fusion. At this point one eye is seen moving out.

2. NPC break (Subjective) – The point where the patient reports he sees double is the subjective break.

3. NPC Recovery (Objective) – The distance at which the patient regains binocular vision. This point is noted as the place where the two eyes realign. The recovery is farther out than the break.

4. NPC Recovery (Subjective) – The distance at which the patient reports that he or she can regain single vision.

6.1 Near point of convergence

The patient wears his near correction. Accommodative targets (reduced Snellen's letters) of different sizes are required. The patient is asked to look at the target, which is shown to him or her from 40 cm. The examiner moves the target towards the patient, while observing his eyes for fixation.

The target is brought towards the patient until he reports doubling (subjective break point) or until the examiner sees one eye lose fixation on the target (objective break point).

Move the target away from the patient, urging him to report when the target appears single again (subjective recovery point) or the examiner notices realignment (objective recovery point).

Record the linear distance from the target to the spectacle plane for both break and recovery points.

Expected findings:

A break point of more than 5 cm is considered abnormal, and the recovery point is required to be within 7 cm.

Procedure in steps:

1. The patient wears his correction for near.

2. An accommodative target (reduced Snellen's letter) is shown to the patient from 40 cm.

3. The patient fixates the target binocularly.

4. Target is brought closer to the patient until he reports doubling or the examiner notices the break in binocular fixation.

5. The linear distance between the target and the spectacle plane is measured. This is the near point of convergence (NPC).

6. The target is then moved away from the patient, until he reports seeing the target single or the examiner notices realignment. This is the recovery point.

7. Break and recovery points are measured and recorded.

A patient may have all the parameters like NPA, NPC, fusional vergences etc. within acceptable limits, but continue to have aesthenopic symptoms. In these cases, it becomes mandatory to check the patient's ability to increase and decrease accommodation binocularly while keeping convergence demand constant. Under these conditions, changes in accommodative convergence are compensated by fusional vergence. Analysis of negative and positive relative accommodation play an important role in determining presbyopic addition too.

6.2 Horizontal fusional vergences at distance

To examine horizontal vergences at distance, appropriate distance correction is placed in the trial frame. An isolated letter is exposed on the Snellen's chart, which is one line larger than the patient's best corrected visual acuity in the poorer eye.

Risley prisms or a prism bar is introduced in front of either of the eyes. The patient is required to look at the target (isolated letter on the Snellen's chart) and keep it clear. Inform the patient that prisms in front of his eyes will be changed, which, in turn, will move the target horizontally. The patient is required to keep the target clear and single and report if:

1. The target blurs.

2. The target becomes double and cannot be made single with effort.

To start the test base in prisms are incorporated in front of the eye. Base in prisms is tested before base out prisms as base out prisms affect accommodation and convergence and hence may affect base in prism findings.

The prisms are changed in front of the eye. Amount of prism in front of the eye is noted when the patient reports blur and break points.

After the break point is reached, decrease the prisms in front of the eye and ask the patient to report when he sees the target single. This is the recovery point.

Prism value for blur, break and recovery is noted. The procedure is repeated with base out prisms for distance.

There is no blur point reported for base in vergence testing for distance. This is because with ideal refraction, the accommodation is fully relaxed and there is no further accommodation which could be relaxed with base in prisms. However, if the patient reports a blur with base in prisms, it is indicative of improper refraction (over corrected myopia or under corrected hyperopia). In such a case refraction needs to be repeated.

Findings are recorded for distance testing, indicating the orientation of the prism with the obtained result. If no blur is seen, then an "X" is marked against it.

Expected findings

Morgan's findings for adult, clinical population:

Distance BI: X/7/4

Distance BOUT: 9/19/12

Procedure in steps:

1. A line better than the best corrected distance visual acuity in the poorer eye is isolated.

2. The patient wears his normal correction for distance and Risley prisms are placed in front of either of the eyes.

3. Base in vergences are checked first, by increasing the base in prisms in front of the eye.

4. The patient is asked to report the blur and the break points.

5. The value of prism in front of the eye is recorded.

6. When the break point is recorded, prism in front of the eye is reduced, until the patient reports seeing the target single again.

7. This is recorded as the recovery point.

8. The procedure is repeated for distance with bout prisms.

6.3 Vertical fusional vergences at distance

This test measures patient's vertical fusional vergences at distance. This test is done with base up or base down prisms.

Base down prisms induce supravergence and base up prisms induce infravergence. While testing vertical vergences, only two findings are expected:

1. Break: At this point, the patient cannot maintain binocular single vision as all the vertical vergences have been exhausted.

2. Recovery: After the break point has been reached, the examiner starts reducing the induced prisms until the image appears single once again. This indicates reduction in retinal disparity to a point where the patient accesses the vertical vergence system again.

There is no blur finding for vertical vergence testing as accommodation does not change during vertical vergence movements.

To examine vertical vergences at distance, appropriate distance correction is placed in the trial frame. An isolated letter is exposed on the Snellen's chart, which is one line larger than the patient's best corrected visual acuity in the poorer eye.

Risley prisms or prism bar is introduced in front of either eye. The patient is required to look at the target (isolated letter on the Snellen's chart) and keep it single. Inform the patient that the prism in front of his eye will be changed, which, in turn, will move the target. The patient is required to keep the target single and report if the target becomes double.

Prisms with their base up are increased in front of the right eye until the patient reports a doubling of the image. This is the break point. On reaching the break point, base up prisms in front of the right eye are reduced until the patient reports seeing the target single. This is the recovery point.

Break and recovery points are recorded. The entire procedure is repeated with base down prisms in front of the right eye and the findings recorded.

Expected findings

Break: 3–4 prisms

Recovery: 1.5–2 prisms

Procedure in steps:

1. A line better than the best corrected visual acuity in the poorer eye is isolated.

2. The patient wears his normal correction for distance and prisms are placed in front of the eye.

3. Base up prisms are increased in front of the right eye.

4. The patient is asked to report the break point.

5. Prisms in front of the right eye are recorded.

6. After the break point is recorded, prisms are reduced, until the patient reports seeing single again.

7. This is recorded as the recovery point.

6.4 Horizontal fusional vergences at near

This procedure is like that done at distance. This measures the patient's ability to use horizontal vergence to maintain binocular vision at near distance.

To examine horizontal vergences at near, appropriate near correction is placed in the trial frame. An isolated line is exposed on the near card, which is one line larger than the patient's best corrected near visual acuity in the poorer eye.

A prism bar is introduced in front of the eye as in the procedure for distance. The patient is required to look at the target (isolated line on the near card) and keep it clear and single. Inform the patient that prisms in front of his or her eyes will be changed, which, in turn will move the target horizontally. The patient is required to keep the target clear and single and report if:

1. The target blurs.

2. The target becomes double and cannot be made single with effort.

Prism value in front of the eye is noted when the patient reports blur and break points. After the break point is reached, decrease the prisms in front of the eye and ask the patient to report when he sees the target single. This is the recovery point.

Prism value for blur, break and recovery is noted. The procedure is repeated with base out prisms for near. Findings are recorded for near testing, indicating the orientation of the prism with the obtained result.

Expected findings:

Morgan's findings for adult, clinical population:

Near BI: 13 / 21 / 13

Near BOUT: 17 / 21 / 11

Procedure in steps:

1. A line better than the best corrected near visual acuity in the poorer eye is isolated.

2. Prisms are incorporated in front of the eye as in the distance procedure.

3. Base in vergences are checked first, by increasing the base in prisms in front of the eye.

4. The patient is asked to report the blur and the break points.

5. When the break point is recorded, prism in front of the eye is reduced until the patient reports seeing the target single again.

6. This is recorded as the recovery point.

7. The procedure is repeated for near with bout prisms.

A patient may be symptomatic despite having normal fusional vergences for both distance and near. In such cases, a patient's fusional vergence facility at near should be checked. This tests the ability of the patient's fusional vergence system to respond to disparity changes within a specific time frame.

6.5 Fusional vergence facility at near

To examine fusional vergence facility at near, appropriate near correction is placed in the trial frame. An isolated vertical line is exposed on the near card, which is one line larger than the patient's best corrected near visual acuity in the poorer eye. 12 prisms base out and 3 prisms base in are used to check the facility of vergence.

The patient is asked to report when the target becomes single and clear. The prisms are flipped to 3 prisms base in position as soon as the patient reports clearing with the 12 prisms base out prisms.

The above-mentioned steps are repeated and the number of full cycles are noted in 1 minute. (One full cycle comprises of clearing both base out and base in prisms).

Number of cycles completed in 60 seconds are recorded.

Expected findings

Fusional facility at near: 15 cycles per minute.

Procedure in steps

1. A line better than the best corrected near visual acuity in the poorer eye is isolated.

2. The patient wears his normal correction for near.

3. A flipper with 12 prisms base out on one side and 3 prisms base in on the other side is introduced with the side having 12 prisms base out in front of the eyes.

4. The patient is asked to report as soon as the line appears single and clear.

5. Prisms are flipped to expose both the eyes to 3 prisms base in.

6. This constitutes one full cycle.

7. Number of cycles completed in 1 minute are recorded.

7. Evaluation of accommodation parameters

For a comprehensive binocular vision examination, it is essential to check the amplitude of accommodation, negative and positive relative accommodation and facility of accommodation. These are required as the accommodation convergence mechanism plays a big role in binocular vision. It is necessary to have these parameters within normal ranges to avoid binocular distress leading to aesthenopic symptoms [2–5].

The amplitude of accommodation is age specific and decreases with age. There are several methods to calculate as well as predict the amplitude of accommodation.

Donder's table is a very good reference to predict it.

Hofstetter's formula is another way to predict amplitude of accommodation:

1. Minimum expected amplitude: 15–0.25 (age)

2. Average expected amplitude: 18.5–0.30 (age)

3. Maximum expected amplitude: 25–0.40 (age)

For a person who is 20 years old, according to Hofstetter's formula:

1. minimum expected amplitude: 15–0.25 (20) = 10 D

2. Average expected amplitude: 18.5–0.30 (age) = 12.5 D

3. Maximum expected amplitude: 25–0.40 (age) = 17 D

For comfortable binocular vision, the amplitude of accommodation of the two eyes should be within one diopter of each other.

There are different ways to physically measure the amplitude of accommodation:

1. Push up method

2. Negative lens method

7.1 Amplitude of accommodation: Push up method

This procedure measures the ability of a patient's crystalline lens to change focus when a near stimulus is provided. The patient's distance correction is placed in the trial frame and the eye not being examined is occluded. His attention is directed towards a row of letters on a near card, one line larger than the best corrected near acuity. The patient is instructed to keep the letters clear. The card is slowly moved closer to the patient and the patient is asked to report when he experiences the first sustained blur. The distance between the card and the patient's spectacle plane is measured in centimeters. This measured distance is called the near point of accommodation (NPA).

The linear distance thus measured is converted into diopters to obtain the amplitude of accommodation.

For example, if the near point of accommodation is measured to be 20 cm, then the amplitude of accommodation is 100 / 20 = 5 D.

Amplitude of accommodation is then measured for the other eye too. Push away is an alternative method usually used with young children, who may not understand the concept of blur. In this method, the card is moved away from close to the patient to a distance where the patient reports that the letters become clear for the first time.

NPA is recorded monocularly as well as binocularly, and then converted to the amplitude of accommodation.

Procedure in steps

1. The patient wears his or her usual correction for distance.

2. He is directed to a row of letters on the near card, which is one line larger than the best corrected near acuity.

3. The card is brought closer to the patient, until he or she reports a sustained blur.

4. The distance between the card and the spectacle plane is measured and is called the near point of accommodation.

5. NPA is converted to its dioptric equivalent to give the amplitude of accommodation.

7.2 Amplitude of accommodation: Minus lens to blur

This is a monocular method to measure the amplitude of accommodation. Minus lenses are used in this test to stimulate accommodation.

Distance prescription is placed in the trial frame and a near card is introduced at 40 cm. The fellow eye is occluded. The patient is asked to look at the line of letters which is one point larger than his near visual acuity.

Minus lenses are added – 0.25 D at a time, with the patient given enough time to clear the letters. Lenses are added until the patient reports first sustained blur. Minus lenses added over the distance prescription plus 2.50 D (accommodative demand for the distance of 40 cm) is the amplitude of accommodation. For example, if – 4.00 D is added over the distance prescription to obtain first sustained blur, then the amplitude of accommodation is 4.00 + 2.50 = 6.50 D.

Procedure is repeated for the other eye and the readings recorded. The amplitude of accommodation as determined by minus lens method is almost 2.0 D less than that measured by the push up method described previously.

Procedure in steps:

1. The patient wears his usual correction for distance.

2. He is directed to a row of letters on the near card, which is one line larger than the best corrected near acuity.

3. Minus lenses are added 0.25 D at a time until the patient reports first sustained blur.

4. Minus lenses plus 2.50 D, gives the amplitude of accommodation for that eye.

5. The procedure is repeated for the fellow eye and measurements recorded.

7.3 Negative and positive relative accommodation

For a non presbyope, the trial frame should have the best corrected distance prescription, and for a presbyope, it should have the patient's near correction.

A near vision card is placed at 40 cm from the patient's spectacle plane. He is required to look at one line larger than his best near visual acuity.

To assess patient's negative relative accommodation (NRA), plus lenses are added binocularly, in steps of +0.25 D. Plus lenses are added until the patient reports first sustained blur. Plus lenses added are noted and this is the NRA value.

Remove the plus lenses until the initial stage of the test is reached (best corrected distance or near correction). On reaching this stage, positive relative accommodation test (PRA) is performed by adding minus lenses binocularly, in steps of – 0.25 D. These are added until the patient reports first sustained blur. Record the total minus lenses added, and this is PRA.

In this test, accommodation is relaxed during NRA and stimulated during PRA. As the test distance is kept constant (40 cm), no accommodative convergence takes place, and that is compensated by changes in fusional vergence.

Expected findings:

For a non presbyope: NRA: + 2.00 D (+/– 0.50 D); PRA: – 2.37D (+/– 1.00 D). For a presbyope, the values vary widely.

Procedure in steps:

1. The patient wears his correction for distance (non presbyope) or near correction (presbyope).

2. He is directed to a row of letters on the near card, which is one line larger than the best corrected near acuity.

3. The patient fixates the target binocularly.

4. Plus lenses are added in +0.25 D steps, until he reports first sustained blur (NRA).

5. Plus lenses are removed slowly and minus lenses are added in - 0.25 D steps until first sustained blur is reported by the patient (PRA).

6. These values are recorded.

To assess the dynamics of accommodative system over a period, accommodative facility testing is done. Patient's ability to make rapid repetitive accommodative changes over an extended period is assessed. This is also known as the inertia of accommodation. Sustenance of accommodation could also be checked while doing this test.

7.4 Accommodative facility

This test is performed both monocularly and binocularly. Monocular test is purely accommodative, while the binocular test is an interaction between accommodation and vergence mechanism.

The patient wears his correction for distance and is required to look at the near card held at 40 cm. A line of letters one line larger than his best near visual acuity is isolated. Plus lenses of +/− 2.00 D flipper is introduced in front of the patient's right eye, while the other eye is occluded. The patient is asked to report as soon as the line of letters clears out. The flipper is flipped to minus lenses and the procedure is continued for 1 minute. Clearing the target through a plus and a minus lens constitutes 1 cycle. Number of cycles performed in 1 minute are recorded. The procedure is repeated for the left eye.

For binocular assessment, flipper is introduced binocularly, and the number of cycles performed in 1 minute is recorded.

Expected findings:

Children (8 to 12 years): 5 cpm binocular, 7 cpm monocular.

Adults (up to 35 years): 10 cpm binocular, 11 cpm monocular.

Monocular findings should be within 4 cpm of each other for each eye.

Procedure in steps:

1. The patient wears his distance correction.

2. He is directed to a row of letters on the near card, which is one line larger than his best corrected near acuity.

3. The patient fixates the target monocularly.

4. A +/− 2.00 D flipper is introduced, and the patient is asked to report as soon as the target clears out.

5. Clearance of target through a plus and a minus lens constitutes 1 cycle.

6. The number of cycles performed in 1 minute is recorded.

7. Procedure is repeated for the other eye and also performed binocularly.

8. Classification of neuromuscular ocular disorders

Nonalignment of visual axes relative to each other is the most common neuromuscular ocular disorders. These are classified based on different criteria [3, 4]:

1. Tropia/phoria

2. Direction of deviation

3. Comitancy

4. Constancy

5. Vergence system

6. Fixation

7. Onset

8.1 Non strabismic binocular vision disorders

These are highly prevalent conditions, next in prevalence only to refractive errors. Patients suffering from these disorders usually present with the following symptoms:

Eyestrain
Diplopia
Headaches
Sleepiness
Blur
Tearing
Inability to change focus from distance to near or vice versa
Lack of attentiveness

To diagnose these problems, evaluation of binocular status as well as accommodation status is required.

Tests required for binocular status evaluation are:

Near point of convergence
Cover test for both distance and near
AC/A ratio
Vergence testing for distance and near
Vergence facility
Randot Stereopsis

Test required for accommodative status evaluation are:
Accommodative amplitude
Accommodative facility
MEM retinoscopy
NRA/PRA
All the above tests can be grouped into 3 basic categories:

1. Positive fusional vergence (PFV)

2. Negative fusional vergence (NFV)

3. Accommodation

For positive fusional vergence group (PFV), following direct and indirect tests need to be performed:
Step vergence / smooth vergence (phoropter)
Vergence facility
NRA
Binocular accommodative facility with plus
NPC
MEM retinoscopy
For negative fusional vergence group (NFV), following direct and indirect tests need to be performed:
Step vergence/smooth vergence (phoropter)
Vergence facility
RA
Binocular accommodative facility with minus
MEM retinoscopy
For accommodative group, following direct and indirect tests need to be performed:
Amplitude of accommodation
Monocular accommodative facility
MEM
Binocular Accommodative Facility.
NRA/PRA.

After performing the above mentioned tests, different syndromes are identified and managed accordingly:

1. Convergence insufficiency

2. Convergence excess

3. Fusional vergence dysfunction

4. Divergence excess

5. Basic Exophoria

6. Divergence Insufficiency

7. Basic Esophoria

8. Vertical Heterophoria

9. Accommodative insufficiency

    a. ill-sustained accommodation

10. Accommodative excess

11. Accommodative infacility

Author details

Aditya Goyal
Sankara College of Optometry, Sankara Eye Foundation, Bangalore, India

*Address all correspondence to: adityagoyal@hotmail.com

References

[1] Borden JA. Burian-von Noorden's binocular vision and ocular motility. Theory and Management of Strabismus. 6th ed. St. Louis, USA: C. V. Mosby

[2] Carlson N, Kurtz D. Clinical Procedures for Ocular Examination. 3rd ed. New York, USA: McGraw Hill

[3] Goss DA. Ocular Accommodation, Convergence, and Fixation Disparity. 3rd ed. UK: Butterworth-Heinemann

[4] Grosvenor T. Primary Care Optometry. 5th ed. UK: Butterworth-Heinemann

[5] Boyd Eskridge J, et al. Clinical Procedures in Optometry. Philadelphia, USA: J. B. Lippincott

Chapter 3

Esodeviations and Associated Syndromes

Fahd Kamal Akhtar

Abstract

Esodeviations refer to misalignments where one or both eyes are turned toward the nose. Various factors contribute to this misalignment, such as disorders in horizontal rectus muscles, refractive errors, and accommodative convergence. The classification of esotropia is based on manifestations, accommodation issues, and consistency with gazes. Latent deviations, termed esophoria, arise due to weak fusional amplitudes and become apparent when fusion is disrupted. Intermittent esotropias manifest under stress or fatigue. Constant esotropias are categorized by comitance, with comitant esotropias involving constant deviation in all gaze directions, likely caused by refractive or accommodative problems. Incomitant esotropias, prevalent in lateral rectus paralysis or medial rectus entrapment, also occur in conditions such as Duane's retraction syndrome, Mobius syndrome, and heavy eye syndrome. Abducent Nerve Palsy arises from damage or dysfunction of the sixth cranial nerve, leading to weakness or paralysis of the lateral rectus muscle. Duane syndrome, a congenital eye movement disorder, restricts eye movement, especially outward, and Moebius syndrome, a rare congenital disorder affecting cranial nerves, results in difficulties with eye coordination. Treatment for esodeviations varies based on the underlying cause and severity, including options such as vision therapy, glasses, prisms, botulinum toxin injections, or surgery to correct muscle imbalances and enhance eye alignment.

Keywords: esodeviation, esophoria, lateral rectus, abducens nerve, strabismus, sixth cranial nerve, esotropia, squint, recession, resection, transposition, Duane

1. Introduction

Esodeviations are the misalignments, in which one or both eyes are positioned towards the nose. Esodeviations are the most common childhood strabismus and equally prevalent to the exodeviations in adults. A lot of factors are responsible for the misalignment of eyes, which include horizontal rectus muscles disorders [1], refractive errors, accommodative convergence etc. The risk factors include hyperopia, anisometropia, low birth weight, prematurity, neural developmental impairment [2].

Esotropia can be classified on the basis of manifestation, accommodation problems and consistency with gazes. The deviation may be manifest or latent. The latent deviations are known as the esophoria, while manifest deviations are known as esotropia, which are further classified as constant or intermittent, comitant or incomitant esotropias.

Esophorias are latent esodeviations, which are caused by weak fusional amplitudes and become prominent as fusion is break under cover. Intermittent esotropias, on the other hand, include the esodeviations which become manifest during stress or fatigue.

Constant esotropias are further grouped on the basis of comitance. In comitant esotropias both eyes remain constantly deviated to each other's in all gaze directions, these are most likely due to refractive or accommodative problems. While incomitant esotropias are present mostly in lateral rectus paralysis or medial rectus entrapment in medial orbital wall fractures [3]. The other causes of incomitant esotropia include syndromes like, Duane's retraction syndrome, Mobius syndrome, heavy eye syndrome etc.

Treatment of esotropia include refractive correction, convergence exercises and muscle surgery.

2. Esophoria

As fusion controls the alignment and keeps the eyes straight with binocular single vision. Sometimes the fusional amplitudes are not much strong to keep eye aligned as fusion breaks. Esophoria is the latent esodeviation that affects eye coordination. Due to insufficient fusional amplitudes, the covered eye tends to deviate nasally as fusion is broken by cover or both eyes focus on different objects.

2.1 Treatment

- Refractive correction
- Prisms; Temporary stick-on Fresnel prisms or spectacles incorporated, maximally 10Δ–12Δ split between both eyes.
- Surgery; occasionally for large esophorias.

3. Comitant esotropias

These are manifest esodeviations in which the angle of deviation remains constant in all directions of gaze. A variety of comitant esotropic deviations are known.

3.1 Essential infantile esotropia

- Manifest by 6 months of age (**Figure 1**)
- Large esodeviation >40Δ–50 Δ (**Figure 2**)
- Equal at distance & near
- Normal to age refractive error (hypermetropic)

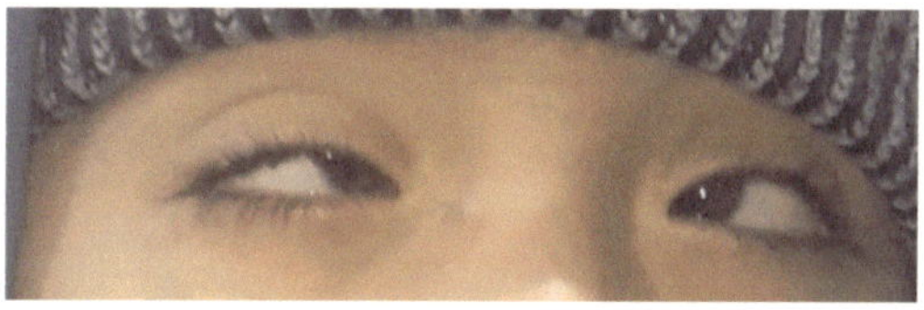

Figure 1.
Infantile esotropia in a 4-month-old child.

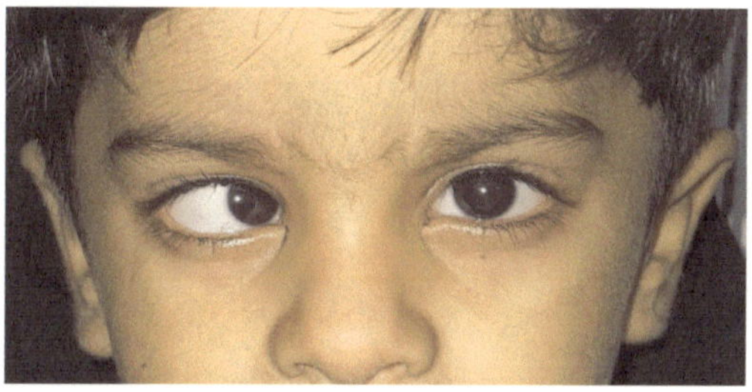

Figure 2.
Infantile esotropia in a 2-year-old child, presented late in a screening clinic.

- Cross fixation is common.
- Amblyopia is uncommon.
- Prohibits fusion and binocular vision.
- Inferior oblique overaction
- Latent nystagmus
- Dissociated vertical deviation may present.

3.1.1 Management

- Cycloplegic refraction to rule out refractive causes.
- Early bilateral medial rectus recession

3.2 Acquired nonaccommodative esotropia

- Develops after 6 months of age (**Figure 3**).
- Esodeviation not corrected by convex lenses (**Figure 4**).
- Starts as intermittent, became as constant.

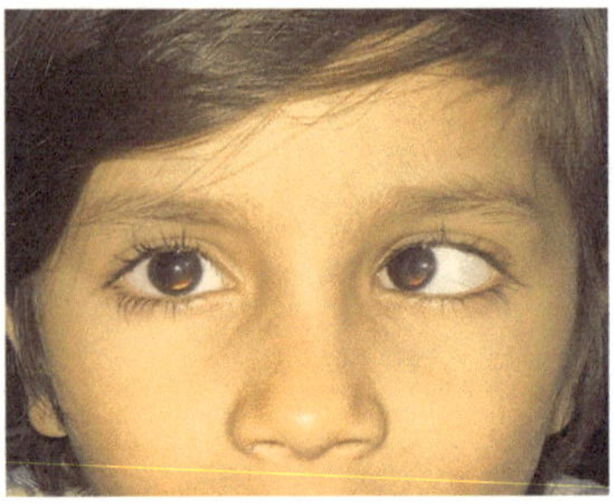

Figure 3.
Acquired non-accommodative esotropia, patient dilated for cycloplegic refraction.

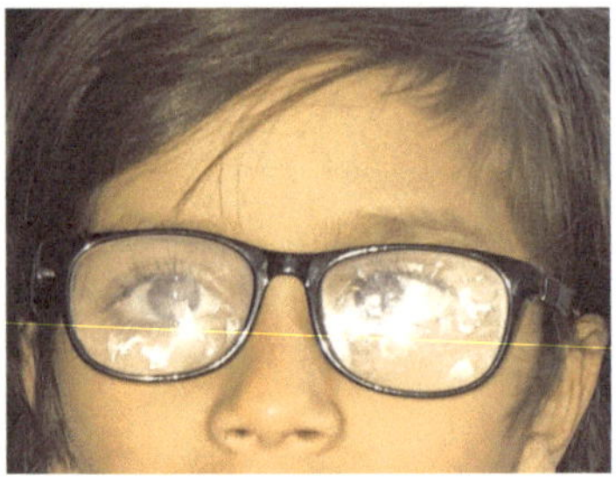

Figure 4.
Refractive correction not effective.

- Small esodeviation, 20Δ–35Δ
- Diplopia may present.

3.2.1 Management

- Bilateral medial rectus recession
- In children <6 years, MRI brain must be done to exclude posterior fossa pathology [4].

3.3 Accommodative esotropia

It is the esodeviation which is associated with the activation of near or accommodative reflex. In accommodation eyes focus on near objects by increasing the curvature of crystalline lens, known as accommodation power (A) and simultaneously converge to focus on object of interest, known as accommodation convergence (AC). Abnormalities in AC/A ratio causes accommodative type of esodeviation. It may present between 6 months and 6 years of age (mean 2½ years). It is further classified into;

3.3.1 Refractive accommodative esotropia

- Mostly present between 1½ year and 3 years (**Figures** 5 and **6**)

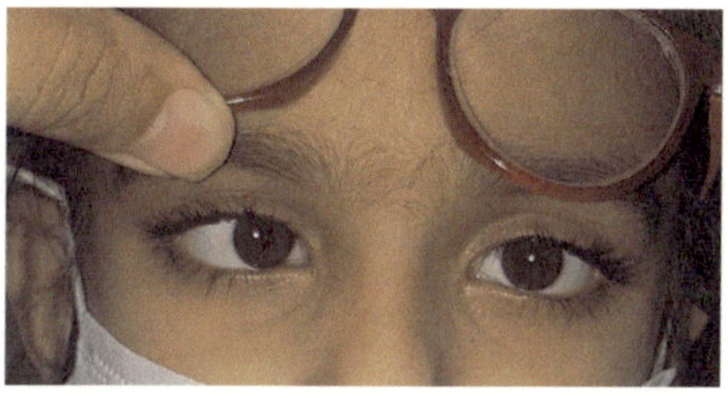

Figure 5.
Refractive accommodative esotropia.

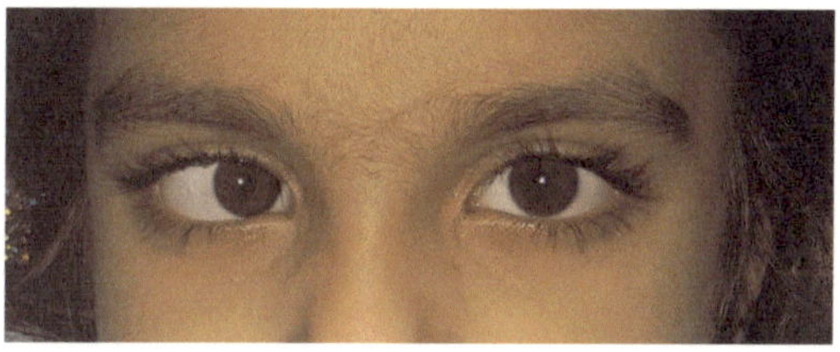

Figure 6.
Refractive accommodative esotropia.

- AC/A ratio is normal
- Excessive hyperopia +2.0D - +10.0D, which cause
- High accommodation convergence (beyond fusional amplitude)
- Small esodeviation 20Δ–30Δ (**Figures 5** and **6**)
- Amblyopia may present

3.3.1.1 Fully accommodative esotropia

- Can be fully aligned by hyperopic correction (**Figure 7**)
- BSV is present

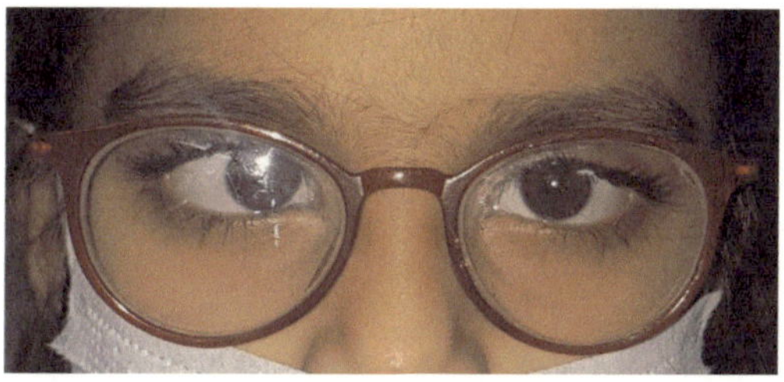

Figure 7.
Fully accommodative esotropia, orthophoric with refractive correction.

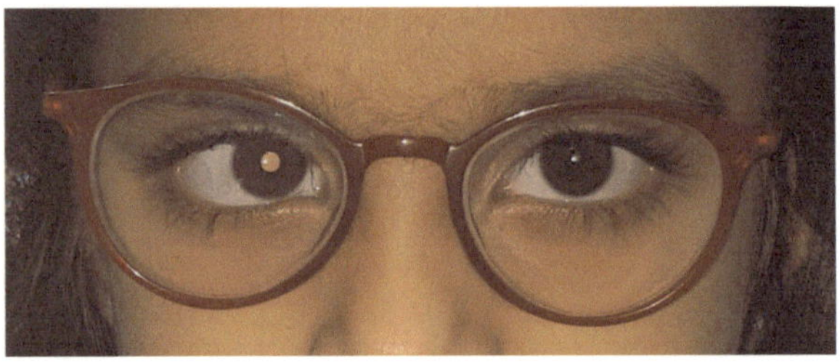

Figure 8.
Partially accommodative esotropia, lessen with refractive correction.

3.3.1.2 Partially accommodative esotropia

- Deviation is reduced but not fully corrected by refraction (**Figure 8**)
- Amblyopia is common as suppression of squinting eye
- ARC may occur
- Surgical correction is usually performed on squinting or amblyopic eye

3.3.2 Non-refractive accommodative esotropia

- High AC/A ratio
- Independent of refractive error (hyperopia and myopia) but hyperopia is frequent
- Straight eyes for distance (with BSV)
- Esotropia for near, suppression is usually present in squinted eye

3.3.2.1 Convergence excess

- Increased accommodation convergence (AC) with normal accommodation (A)
- Near point of accommodation is normal
- Orthophoric with bifocals, executive type is preferred
- Bilateral medial rectus is performed

3.3.2.2 Hypo-accommodative convergence excess

- Normal accommodation convergence (AC) with decreased accommodation (A)
- Near point of accommodation is remote
- Executive type bifocals may be advised for near work
- Surgical correction may be considered only when refractive correction is not sufficient.

3.4 Non-accommodative convergence excess/near esotropia

- Presents in young adults and older children (**Figure 9**)
- Esotropia for near
- Orthophoric/small esophoria with BSV for distance
- Non-significant refractive error (**Figure 10**)
- Normal or low AC/A ratio
- Near point of accommodation is normal

3.4.1 Treatment

Bilateral medial rectus recessions.

3.5 Distance esotropia

- Presents in myopic healthy young adults
- Esotropia for distance, may be intermittent
- Orthophoric for near
- Normal bilateral abduction

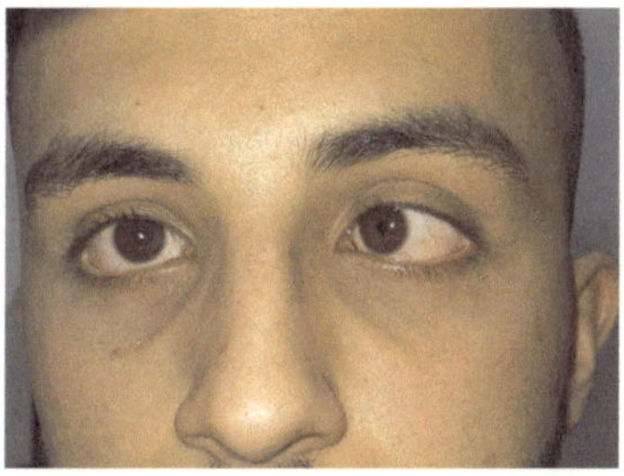

Figure 9.
Non-accommodative convergence excess esotropia.

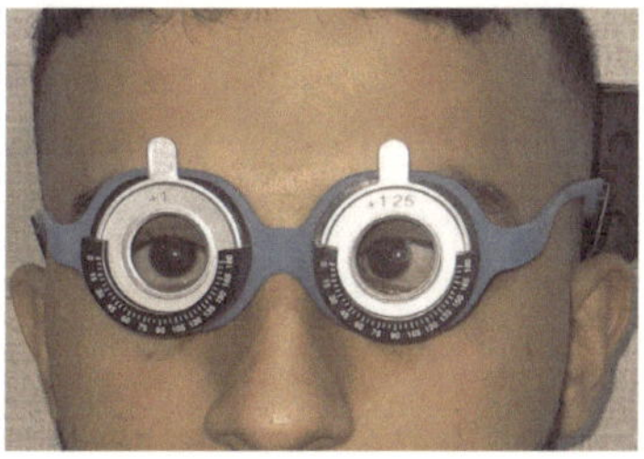

Figure 10.
Non-significant refractive error, which is also not correcting esotropia.

- Reduced fusional divergence amplitudes
- No neurological deficit

3.5.1 Treatment

- Prisms until spontaneous resolution
- Surgery if persists

3.6 Acute esotropia/late-onset esotropia

- Presents usually around 5 years–6 years of age but in young adults too
- Sudden onset of esotropia and diplopia (**Figure 11**).
- Non-significant refractive error
- Normal ocular motility
- Underlying neurological disorder may present

3.6.1 Management

- Cranial nerve examination
- Pupil reflexes
- Fundus examination for optic disc pathology
- Re-establishing BSV
- Prevent suppression

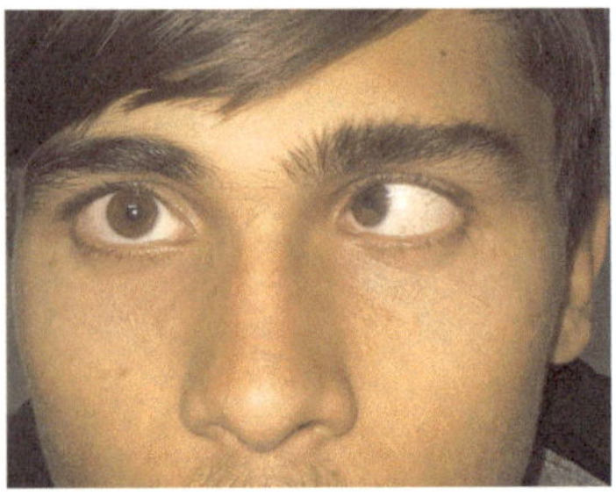

Figure 11.
Acute onset esotropia in 17-year-old male with history of sudden onset of diplopia 2 weeks ago. Fundus examination reveals bilateral disc swelling.

3.6.2 Treatment

- Prisms with glasses
- Botulinum toxin in medial rectus
- Strabismus correction surgery

3.7 Sensory-deprivation esotropia

In children younger than 4 years of age, many organic conditions cause impaired focusing to light to retina and perception by the visual cortex, thus hindring the fusion development. This causes the eye to deviate inwards nasally. In older children and adults these cause the sensory exotropia. These conditions may be uniocular or binocular as;

- Uncorrected refractive errors
- Anisometropic hypermetropia
- Severe ptosis (**Figure 12**)
- Buphthalmos
- Corneal opacities
- Congenital corneal dystrophies
- Congenital cataracts
- PHPV and persistent fetal vasculature
- Retinopathy of prematurity
- Retinal and optic disc colobomas
- Retinal detachments
- Macular dystrophies
- Retinoblastoma
- Coats disease
- Optic nerve anomalies etc.

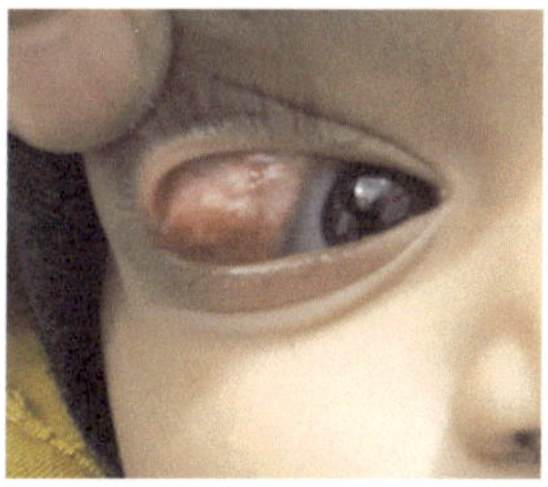

Figure 12.
Sensory-deprivation esotropia due to severe ptosis secondary to lid hemangioma in 8 months old child.

3.7.1 Treatment

- Dilating fundus examination to establish the cause.
- Treating the underlying cause first.
- Amblyopia therapy
- Cosmetic strabismus correction

3.8 Consecutive esotropia

Consecutive esotropia is said when an exotropic person becomes esotropic. It is usually caused by the surgical correction of exotropia, with incidence rate reported between 6 and 20%. The factors involve in the overcorrection of divergent squints;

- Poor vision
- Congenital retinal or optic nerve anomalies
- Intermittent distance exotropia (IDEX)

3.8.1 Treatment

- Comitant small deviation (10Δ–15Δ) should be observe for 2 weeks for spontaneous resolution.
- Re-do strabismus correction by medial rectus recession or lateral rectus advancement in patients with good vision.
- Repeated botulinum toxin injections in medial rectus muscle is preferred in patients with poor vision.

3.9 Divergence insufficiency

- Common in elderly patients
- Esotropia; distance fixation > near fixation
- Diagnosis of exclusion
- Caused by the weakening or rupturing of connective tissue between lateral rectus muscle and superior rectus muscle, causing sagging of lateral rectus muscle [5].
- Associated with neurologic trauma, pontine tumors, raised intracranial pressure.

3.9.1 Management

- Spontaneous resolution
- Base out prisms in glasses.

3.10 Cyclic esotropia

It is a rare condition which is mostly characterized by esotropia lasting for 24 hours alternating with 24 hours of orthophoria. The incidence is 1 in every 3000–5000 patients. Cyclic esotropia may persist for months or years until it develops into a constant esotropia.

3.10.1 Treatment

Both eyes medial rectus recession has good results. Measurement is done on the basis of photographic evidence or the orthoptic assessment during the esotropic cycle, or until the esotropia becomes constant.

4. Incomitant esodeviations

In contrast to the comitant esodeviations, in which the degree of deviation remains constant in all directions of gazes, angle of deviation increases in lateral gaze while fixating distantly in incomitant esodeviation. Incomitant esodeviations are caused by;

4.1 Central nervous system pathologies

- Increased intracranial pressure
- Acquired sixth nerve palsy

4.2 Medial rectus restriction

- Thyroid eye disease
- Muscle entrapment in medial orbital wall fracture

4.3 Lateral rectus weakness

- Isolated sixth nerve palsy
- Slipped/detached lateral rectus muscle from trauma/surgery.

5. Abducens nerve palsy

Abducens Nerve is the Sixth Cranial nerve and responsible for the movement of the Lateral rectus nerve. The sixth nerve palsy is the most common extraocular muscle palsy in adults and second most common in children.

5.1 Presentation

- Convergent squint due to unopposed action of antagonist Medial rectus

- The esotropia is incomitant, greater in looking towards affected gaze and more at fixing distance than near.
- Diplopia; binocular and horizontal, worsen for distant vision and in direction of paretic muscle.

5.2 Etiology

As the abducens nerve has the longest intracranial course among all cranial nerves, hence it is more prone to the damage.

In children the causes of palsy include,

- Congenital [6]
  - Associated with birth trauma,
  - Hydrocephalus
  - Cerebral palsy,
- Acquired [7]
  - Tumor,
  - Trauma,
  - Inflammation,
  - Infection
  - Idiopathic.

In adults the causes of the sixth nerve palsy are divided into [8].

- Common causes
  - Vasculopathies due to microvascular ischemia,
  - Trauma (**Figure 13**)
  - Idiopathic
- Other causes include:
  - Stroke
  - Multiple sclerosis,
  - Raised intracranial pressure,

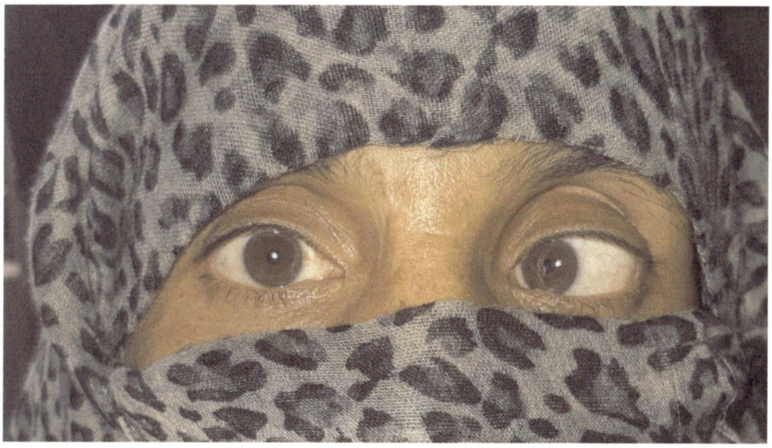

Figure 13.
Traumatic left sixth nerve palsy in 45-year-old female.

- Cavernous sinus mass; aneurysm, meningioma, tumor metastasis
- Sarcoidosis
- Vasculitis
- Lymes disease
- Neurosyphilis

5.3 Differential diagnosis

The differentials of limited abduction involve:

5.3.1 Thyroid eye disease

- Proptosis (**Figure 14**) [8]
- Lid Retraction
- Lid Lag
- Injection over involved rectus
- Positive FDT (Forced Duction Test)

5.3.2 Myasthenia gravis

- Diplopia is fluctuating, variable and fatigable [8].
- Ptosis is common.
- Generalize fatigability may present.

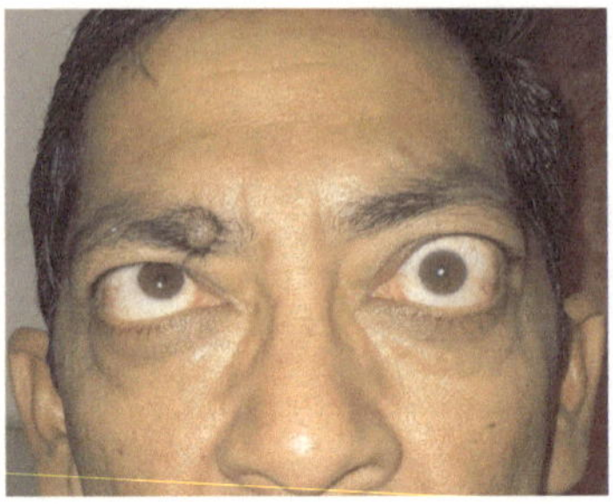

Figure 14.
Esodeviation in thyroid eye disease. Right eye supro-nasal misalignment. Proptosis and lid retraction are also notable in both eyes.

- Shortness of breath and hoarseness
- Positive ice and rest tests

5.3.3 Duane retraction syndrome, type 1

- Congenital
- Narrowing of the palpebral fissure in adduction (**Figure 15**)
- Retraction of globe

5.3.4 Mobius syndrome

- Congenital
- Bilateral facial paralysis

5.3.5 Convergence spasm

- Intermittent, variable convergence
- Miosis
- Deficient Abduction in versions but with full ductions

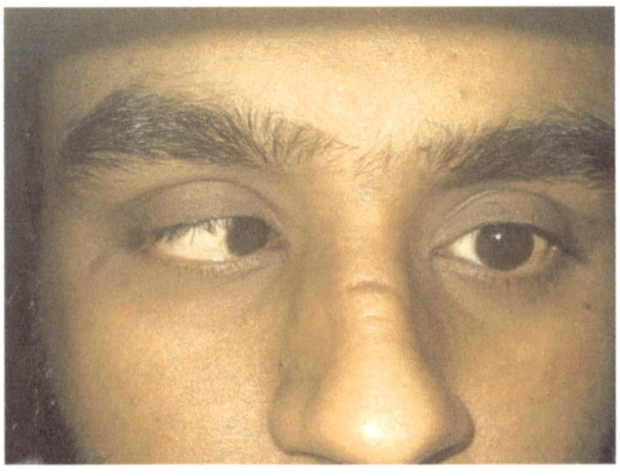

Figure 15.
Duane retraction syndrome, right eye induced ptosis and left eye abduction deficit.

5.3.6 Primary divergence insufficiency

- Acquired
- Esotropia
- Diplopia at distance with binocular single vision (BSV) at near

5.3.7 Giant cell arteritis GCA

- Extraocular muscle ischemia
- Age > 55 years

5.4 Management & work up

5.4.1 Children

- History:
  - Birth trauma,
  - Recent illness,
  - Neurological symptoms,
  - Ear infections
- Complete Ophthalmic & Neurological Examination
- MRI brain

5.4.2 Adults

- History:
  - Onset & progression,
  - Systemic diseases; hypertension, diabetes, thyroid dysfunction,
- Complete Ophthalmic & Neurological Examination:
  - Extraocular movements,
  - Corneal sensation,
  - Fundus examination for optic disc (swelling /papilledema)

- Hess Chart (**Figure 16**)
    - Underation of ipsilateral lateral rectus muscle
    - Normal/overaction of contralateral medial rectus muscle
- Systemic Examination; blood pressure,
- Laboratory Examination:
    - Fasting blood sugar
    - HbA1c,
    - Serum lipid profile
    - ESR
    - CRP
    - CSF analysis
    - Lyme antibody titer
    - FTA-ABS or treponemal-specific assay, VDRL or RPR

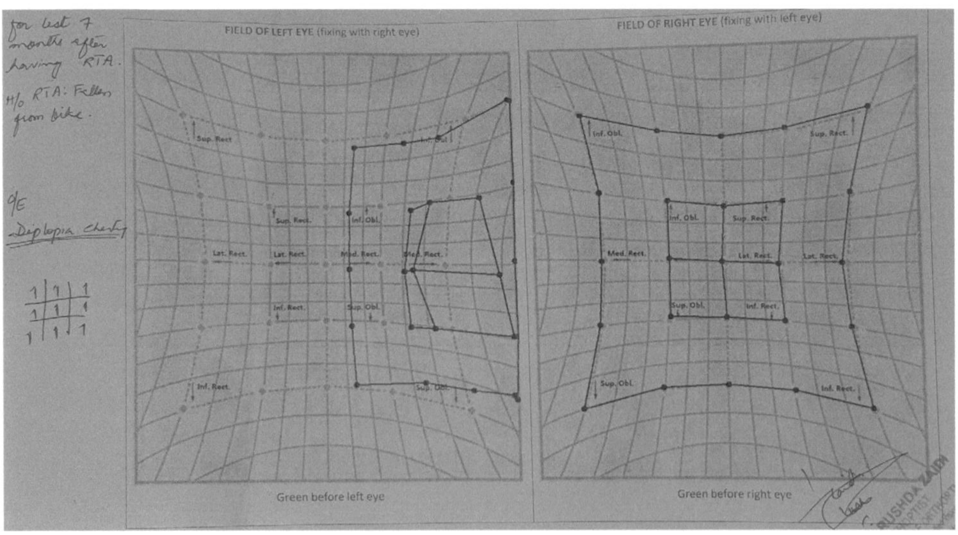

Figure 16.
Hess chart of 45-year-old patient, with history of road traffic accident 8 month ago, showing left lateral rectus under-action. Medial rectus muscles of both eyes showing no overaction. Due to compensatory head posture towards left the patient has no complaint of diplopia.

- MRI Brain
  - In all patients younger than 45 years,
  - Non-isolated sixth nerve lesion,
  - History of neoplasms,
  - Patients without microvascular diseases.
  - Papilledema

5.5 General treatment

- Treat the underlying etiology.
- Abducens nerve palsy due to microvascular causes are observed as they recover within 3 to 6 months.
- Diplopia is managed by [9].
  - Occlusion; Bangerter filter, eye patch, central glass patch. It eliminates confusion and diplopia, prevents suppression and amblyopia, and minimizes contracture of ipsilateral medial rectus. In patients <10 years, patching is avoided due to high risks of amblyopia.
  - Base-out Fresnel or ground in prisms. Limited role in maintaining BSV as the deviation is incomitant.
- Botulinum Toxin: it is injected into medial rectus to prevent secondary contracture and to weak medial rectus in transposition procedures.
- Surgical intervention is advised only in patients having stable deviations for at least 6 months.
- Follow up every 6 weeks until the resolution of palsy or stabilization of deviation.

5.6 Surgical management

5.6.1 Aim

Surgical correction is always planned for realignment of the globe in primary position [10].

5.6.2 Surgical protocols

Surgical management of the Lateral Rectus disorder in patients having stable orthoptic measurements for more than 6 months, depends upon [11];

- Medial rectus fibrosis
- Lateral rectus residual function

For medial rectus fibrosis, forced duction test is performed. If FDT is positive that shows tight medial rectus, recession of the medial rectus is done (**Figure 17**).

For lateral rectus, active force generation test (FGT) is performed.

- Active FGT present; Resection of LR
- Active FGT absent; transposition procedures

If lateral rectus shows any residual function, then recession of ipsilateral MR along with supra-maximum (12–14 mm) resection of lateral rectus is performed.

5.7 Transposition surgeries for lateral rectus muscle palsy

When there is no LR function on active FGT, a variety of transposition surgeries can be planned for realigning the eyes in primary position, these include; (**Figure 18**).

5.7.1 Full tendon transposition

Disinsertion of full width tendons of superior and inferior recti and transposing them towards lateral rectus insertion [12]. This procedure has risk of anterior segment ischemia which can be minimized by conserving muscular branches of anterior ciliary artery, and avoiding extensive dissection (**Figure 18A**).

5.7.2 Cross-adjustable technique

To increase the effectiveness of the full tendon transposition by increasing path length to avoid the resection of vertical rectus muscles, the tendons are passed beneath the LR tendon and attached at the opposite corners of LR Insertion [13]. This technique also decreases the need of ipsilateral MR recession in many cases (**Figure 18B**).

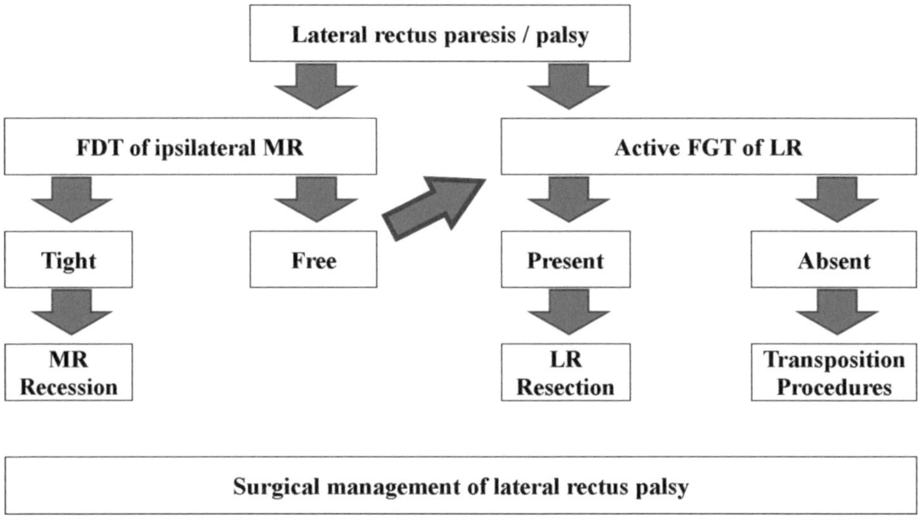

Figure 17.
Surgical management for lateral rectus palsy, based on the standard treatment protocol described by American Academy of ophthalmology.

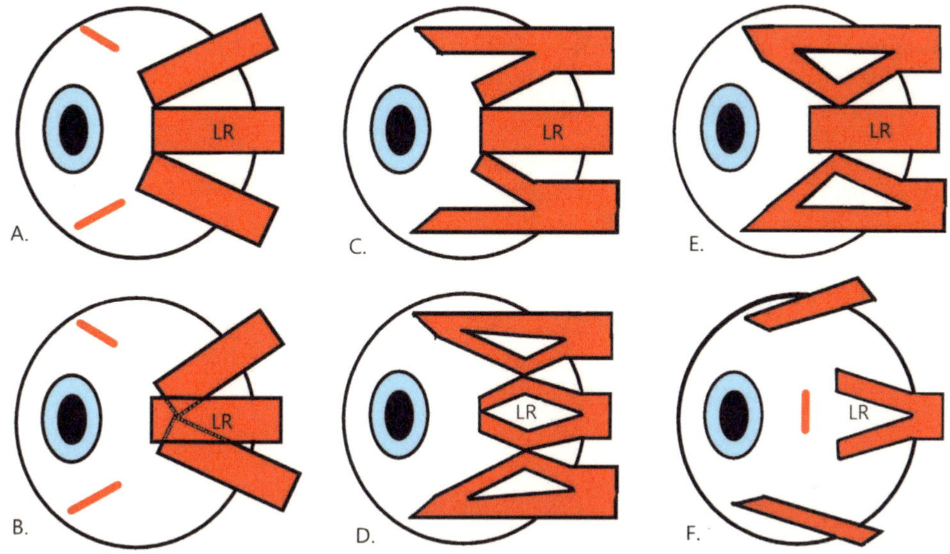

Figure 18.
Diagrammatic presentation of surgeries to treat lateral rectus palsy/disorders. A. Full tendon transposition; B. Full tendon transposition with cross-adjustable technique; C. Hummelsheim procedure; D. Jensen's procedure; E. Nishida's procedure; F. LR recession with possible Y-splitting for treating leash phenomenon in Duane's retraction syndrome.

5.7.3 Hummelsheim

Vertical recti are split half tendon width up to 14 mm approximately from the insertion. The temporal halves of superior and inferior recti are disinserted and transposed to the lateral rectus insertion [14]. Care must be taken to preserve the anterior ciliary vessels during procedure (**Figure 18C**).

5.7.4 Augmented/modified Hummelsheim

Transposed half tendons are further resected to increase the effectiveness of Hummelsheim procedure along with medial rectus recession. It is reported to correct deviation up to $40\Delta \pm 5\Delta$ [15].

5.7.5 Jensen's procedure

First described by Jensen et al. in 1964 [16], the bellies of superior and inferior recti are split half tendon width and tied to lateral rectus muscle without disinsertion, 12–14 mm behind from the insertion with non-absorbable suture (**Figure 18D**). To avoid anterior segment ischemia, at least one ciliary artery must be protected. In vessel sparing modification of Jensen's procedure, the split muscles are stitched together by looping stitch underneath the vessels.

5.7.6 Nishida's procedure

This procedure was described by Nishida et al. in 2003 [17]. In this technique the vertical rectus muscles are exposed by limbal based peritomy. After dissecting intermuscular septum along lateral margin of each muscle, vertical recti are split half tendon width up to 15 mm from the insertion. With 6–0 nylon sutures, lateral half of each muscle is secured at 8–10 mm from the insertion and anchored at 8 mm posterior to LR insertion to sclera (**Figure 18E**).

5.7.7 Superior rectus transposition

Jhonston et al. described transposition of the superior rectus muscle only to the lateral rectus insertion [18]. It was postulated to prevent anterior segment ischemia and to simplify the procedure. The procedure improves esotropia, abduction and head turn with minimal vertical misalignment.

5.7.8 Inferior rectus transposition

Alternative to superior rectus transposition, this procedure is helpful to improve esotropia, abduction limitation and head turn, along with the correction of hypertropia [19].

5.8 Follow up

Postoperatively, patients should be managed under close observation. Prisms should be prescribed for any residual diplopia. Since there are increased chances of anterior segment ischemia in the first 6 months of the primary surgery, hence the repeat surgery should always be planned after 6 months of primary surgery, providing the ample time for collaterals to develop.

5.9 Surgical complication

- Anterior segment ischemia [20]
- Under correction; of primary esotropia and head posture
- Over correction; consecutive exotropia
- Diplopia
- Induced vertical deviations [21].
- Conjunctival cyst
- Conjunctival prolapse.
- Corneal dellen
- Tenon's prolapse.

- Scleral perforation
- Lost/Slipped Muscle
- Bradycardia
- Secondary infections.

5.10 Prognosis

Rush JA reported an overall recovery rate of 49.6%, with 71% recovery in patients with systemic diseases (diabetes mellitus, hypertension, atherosclerosis etc.) [22].

6. Duane syndrome

It is also known as Stilling-Turk-Duane syndrome. Duane syndrome was first described in 1905 by Alexander Duane [23]. It is congenital, non-progressive syndrome [24] characterized by some or all of the following:

- Abduction limitation, usually complete (**Figure 19**)
- Globe retraction on attempted adduction
- Induced Ptosis; narrowing of palpebral fissure on adduction (**Figure 19**).
- Adduction limitation, usually partial [25]
- Oblique movement on attempted adduction
- Leash Phenomenon, Upshoot or downshoot of globe with adduction
- Widening of palpebral aperture on abduction
- Convergence insufficiency

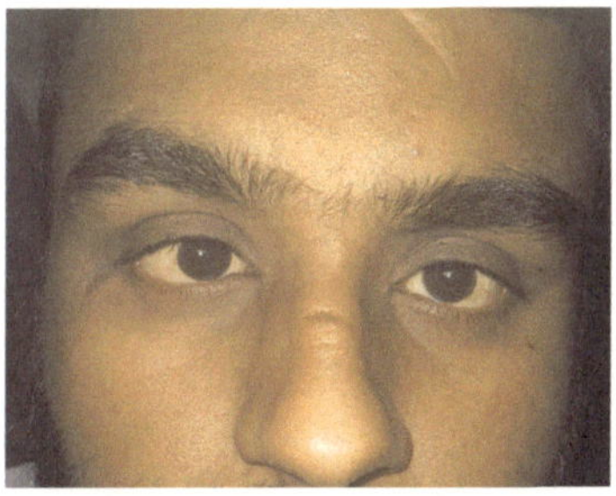

Figure 19.
Duane type 1, right small angle esotropia in primary gaze.

6.1 Types

Duane retraction syndrome is divided into three types with multiple subgroups; the difference in clinical features are;

6.1.1 Type 1

- 75–80% of patients [26]
- Esotropia in primary gaze (**Figure 19**)
- Compensatory head turn to the involved side.

6.1.2 Type 2

- 5–10% of patients [26]
- Exotropia in primary gaze
- Compensatory head turn to the uninvolved side.

6.1.3 Type 3

- 10–20% of patients [26]
- Present with either an esotropia or exotropia in primary gaze
- Compensatory head turn to the involved side
- The ability to adduct in this type is absent to restricted as compared to normal to mildly restricted in types 1 and 2.

6.2 Etiology

- About 90% of the cases are sporadic and commonly unilateral [27].
- Remaining 10% cases are bilateral and inherited [27]:
    - Type 1: Autosomal Dominant (locus 8q13) [24]
    - Type 2: Autosomal Dominant (CHN1 gene mutation at DURS 2 locus 2q31-q32.1) [24] & Autosomal recessive [28]

6.3 Pathophysiology

Duane syndrome results from aberrant lateral rectus innervation by third nerve as abducens motor neurons are absent or dysplastic.

6.3.1 Myogenic theory

It suggests that lateral rectus is fibrosed or inelastic and medial rectus has abnormal far posterior insertion [26].

6.3.2 Neurogenic theory

It was suggested by postmortem studies at John Hopkins University in 1980 [29]. At 4–8 weeks of gestation, a disturbance in embryologic development results in abducens nerve absent which causes aberrant lateral rectus innervation by third nerve [29]. Hence both MR & LR are innervated by oculomotor nerve, their simultaneous activation results in globe retraction [30].

6.4 Diagnosis

Duane syndrome is diagnosed primarily based on clinical features:

- Paralytic squint: 76% have tropias in primary gaze [24].
- Abduction limitation
- Narrowing of fissure on adduction
- Globe retraction
- Upshoot or downshoot with adduction
- Compensatory head posture
- Good visual Acuity [24]

6.5 Management

6.5.1 Evaluation

- History: onset, trauma, family history, other ocular or systemic diseases [27].
- Complete ophthalmic examination; visual acuity, extraocular movements, aberrant movements and retractions, compensatory head position,
- Systemic examination, cranial nerves evaluation
- Forced duction and active force generation tests to evaluate tight muscles.
- Genetic evaluation and counseling when familial pattern is noted [26].
- MRI brain and orbit, for visualization of anatomy.

6.5.2 Non-surgical management

- Refractive correction by glasses or contact lens [26]
- Corrective prisms for abnormal head posture [26]
- Amblyopia prevention & treatment; new cases must be evaluated 3–6 monthly [26].
- Botulinum Toxin: to minimize leash phenomenon [31].
- Children >7 years with good vision and binocularity can be evaluated annually [26].

6.6 Surgical management

6.6.1 Limitations

- Cannot fully cure the disease.
- Only correct tropias in primary gaze
- Improve head posture.
- Improve leash phenomenon [26]
- Either recessions only or transpositions are done; muscle resections can never be planned.

6.6.2 Indications

- Compensatory head posture (CHP) $\geq 15°$ [32]
- Neck discomfort due to CHP
- Significant tropia, Cosmesis issues [32]
- Severe induced ptosis; PFH $\leq 50\%$ of normal on adduction [33]
- Severe co-contraction [34]

6.6.3 Contraindications

- Orthophoria [33]
- Normal head posture [33]
- Young age [33]

6.6.4 Surgical procedures

A variety of surgeries have been advised depending upon the type and clinical features of the disease.

- DRS type 1 & 3 + face turn

Based on FDT; MR recession only or Transposition of vertical rectus muscles to lateral rectus [35].

- Full tendon transposition of vertical recti (**Figure 18A**).
- Full tendon transposition with cross-adjustable technique
- Jensen's procedure (**Figure 18D**).
- Nishida's procedure (**Figure 18E**).
- Superior rectus transposition
- Inferior Rectus transposition
- DRS type 1 & 3 + Leash phenomenon/severe globe retraction
    - Recession of both MR & LR with possible Y-splitting of LR [26] (**Figure 18F**).
- DRS type 2 + face turn (fixation with uninvolved eye)
    - Ipsilateral LR recession [26]
- DRS type 2 + face turn (fixation with involved eye)
    - Contralateral LR recession [26]
- DRS type 2 + Leash phenomenon
    - Ipsilateral LR recession with possible Y-splitting (**Figure 18F**) [26].

6.6.5 Surgical complications

Under correction; of primary esotropia and head posture [33].
Over correction; consecutive exotropia [33].
Induced vertical deviations; post transposition procedures [33].

7. High myopia esotropia

In patients with high myopia and large axial lengths, tenon muscle pulleys of superior rectus and lateral rectus muscles may become instable. This causes the bulging of globe through the defect of muscle pulleys resulting in inferior displacement of the lateral rectus muscle and nasal displacement of the superior rectus muscle.

7.1 Management

Magnetic resonance imaging (MRI) should be done in every high myope with acquired esotropia to diagnose the condition. The esotropia is treated by repairing muscle pulleys by plication of the superior rectus muscle and lateral rectus muscle with a non-absorbable suture.

8. Moebius syndrome

It is a rare congenital, non-progressive syndrome involving both abducens and facial nerve palsies.

8.1 Clinical features

- It is characterized by;
- Lagophthalmos
- Esotropia
- Limitation in abduction and/or adduction
- Intact vertical movements & bell's phenomenon, saving cornea intact.
- Unilateral/bilateral, partial/complete facial nerve palsy
- Mask like face appearance
- Cranial nerves V, VIII, X & XII may be affected too.
- Tongue atrophy, limbs and chest deformities may occur.

8.2 Management

- No definitive treatment
- Behavioral management; suction aids
- Rehabilitation; Orthopedics surgeons
- Temporary tarsorrhaphy to prevent dry eye.
- Medial rectus recession for esotropia
- Transposition surgeries; inconsistent results

9. Idiopathic orbital inflammatory syndrome

Idiopathic orbital myositis is relatively less common, non-infective, non-granulomatous, non-neoplastic inflammation of isolated or multiple extraocular muscles. Lateral rectus is usually less involved than medial rectus.

9.1 Features

- Tendon involving muscle enlargement.
- Pain, more on eye movements
- Proptosis
- Periorbital edema
- Diplopia

9.2 Management

- Systemic evaluation
- Autoimmune profile (CBC, ESR, ACE, ANA, cANCA, pANCA, LDH)
- Imaging: Orbital MRI with DWI protocol
- Corticosteroids (1 mg/kg/day)
- Low dose radiation
- Steroid sparing agents (methotrexate, cyclophosphamide)

10. Conclusion

Esodeviations involve a variety of disorders which cause eyes to move nasally inwards, the management depends upon addressing these disorders. In general, the management protocol involves;

10.1 Observation and systemic evaluation

Acute onset esodeviations are usually lateral rectus palsies secondary to systemic hypertension, diabetes mellitus, atherosclerosis and benign intracranial hypertension, which are usually self-resolving, subject to the treatment of underlying etiology and any life-threatening condition, if present. Systemic evaluation for the above-mentioned diseases along with the laboratory profiles and radiological imaging are key steps in observing these acute lesions.

In case of trauma involving the sixth nerve, only the emergency traumatic repairs must be performed first. The esotropia associated with traumatic sixth nerve palsy is left observed for at least 6 months before offering any surgical intervention. Non-surgical treatment options must be offered to all patients during the observation to relive diplopia and asthenopia.

10.2 Non-surgical treatment

Non-surgical treatments are aimed to restore vision, relive diplopia and asthenopia. Patching can help to treat amblyopia and minimize diplopia. In children and young adults with esotropias associated with underlying amblyopia, the healthy eye is completely patched to enhance the sensory perception of the lazy eye. While, in elder adults with lateral rectus palsy, patching the center part of glasses helps in minimizing the diplopia in primary gaze with keeping side vision intact. Full refractive correction by hyperopic convex lenses and bifocals helps in treating the accommodative esotropias and convergence excess esotropias respectively. In divergence insufficiency, divergence orthoptic exercises are advised with or without prisms. Prescribing prisms may relieve diplopia well. Prism glasses and Fresnel prisms are tolerated well in patients who are kept under observation before planning any surgical procedure. Medical management is necessary for the esotropia associated with systemic diseases. In addition to the systemic medicines, some of the drugs used are vitamin B12, corticosteroids and disease modifying agents. Corticosteroids by their anti-inflammatory effects are prescribed in thyroid eye disease, myositis and traumatic brain and orbital injuries. Botulinum toxin has gained much popularity for non-surgical chemodenervation of the medial rectus muscle in treating infantile and acute esotropias. It also helps to prevent medial rectus fibrosis in lateral rectus palsy and also help to prevent anterior chamber ischemia by sparing medial rectus recession in transposition procedures.

10.3 Surgical treatment

The main aim of surgical treatment is to attempt in developing a good binocular single vision by restoring the regular alignment of both eyes and addressing any pathology causing sensory deprivation. Treating ptosis, cataract and other causes are sometimes more important than to treat the esotropia alone. In medial rectus muscle entrapments, medial orbital wall is repaired as early as possible to avoid the development of muscle fibrosis and ischemia. in treating abnormal head posture and diplopia, surgical options must be considered to offer, only when there are more than 6 months passed with static orthoptic measurements. It is advised to treat amblyopia prior to surgery but sometimes surgery, itself, is the only option to treat the amblyopia as early as possible, before development of any degeneration at the level of lateral geniculate nucleus. Intermittent esotropias have good surgical prognosis over constant and alternating ones. The typical surgical approach for comitant esotropia is bilateral medial rectus recession or unilateral medial rectus recession and lateral rectus resection (recess-resect procedure). In incomitant esotropias surgical approaches vary with the type of esotropia, as transposition of vertical recti. Different transposition procedures of vertical rectus muscles are done to compensate for the limited abduction. These procedures include full tendon transposition, partial tendon vertical transposition, split muscle transpositions etc. The main complication of these surgeries is the anterior segment ischemia, which can be avoided by preserving muscular arteries during surgery. Other complications include under corrections and induced vertical deviations. Loop myopexy is considered for myopic esotropia /heavy eye syndrome.

Acknowledgements

I would like to acknowledge the motivation given by Dr. Muna Malik, and her help in typing, proofreading and reviewing this manuscript.

The project is not funded by any sponsor and all the expenses were borne by the author himself.

Conflict of interest

The author declares no conflict of interest.

Notes/thanks/other declarations

Thanks to my colleagues and patients who gave me strength to write this chapter.

All pictures are taken with the consent of patients, subjected not to disclose their particulars and full-face identity. The diagrams are made by the author.

Author details

Fahd Kamal Akhtar
Services Hospital, Lahore, Punjab, Pakistan

*Address all correspondence to: fkak82@gmail.com

References

[1] Cabrera AF, Suárez-Quintanilla J. Anatomy, Head and Neck, Eye Lateral Rectus Muscle. Treasure Island (FL): StatPearls Publishing [Internet]; 2022

[2] Bohnsack BL, Gallina D, Thompson H, Kasprick DS, Lucarelli MJ, Dootz G, et al. Development of extraocular muscles requires early signals from periocular neural crest and the developing eye. Archives of Ophthalmology. 2011;**129**(8):1030-1041

[3] Shumway CL, Motlagh M, Wade M. Anatomy, Head and Neck, Eye Extraocular Muscles. Treasure Island (FL): StatPearls Publishing [Internet]; 2021

[4] Liu JK. Combined petrosal approach for resection of a large trigeminal Schwannoma with Meckel's cave involvement-part II: Microsurgical approach and tumor resection: 2-dimensional operative video. Operative Neurosurgery (Hagerstown, Md.). 2021; **20**(3):E226

[5] Chaudhuri Z, Demer JL. Sagging eye syndrome: Connective tissue involution as a cause of horizontal and vertical strabismus in older patients. JAMA Ophthalmology. 2013;**131**(5):619-625

[6] McKay VH, Touil LL, Jenkins D, Fattah AY. Managing the child with a diagnosis of Moebius syndrome: More than meets the eye. Archives of Disease in Childhood. 2016;**101**(9):843-846

[7] Teksam O, Keser AG, Konuskan B, Haliloglu G, Oguz KK, Yalnizoglu D. Acute abducens nerve paralysis in the pediatric emergency department: Analysis of 14 patients. Pediatric Emergency Care. 2016;**32**(5):307-311

[8] Kung NH, Van Stavern GP. Isolated ocular motor nerve palsies. In: Seminars in Neurology. Vol. 35, No. 5. New York, NY, USA: Thieme Medical Publishers; 2015. pp. 539-548

[9] Heckmann JG, Vachalova I, Lang CJ, Pitz S. Neuro-ophthalmology at the bedside: A clinical guide. Journal of Neurosciences in Rural Practice. 2018; **9**(4):561-573

[10] Rosenbaum AL. The efficacy of rectus muscle transposition surgery in esotropic Duane syndrome and VI nerve palsy. Journal of American Association for Pediatric Ophthalmology and Strabismus. 2004;**8**(5):409-419

[11] von Noorden GK. A reassessment of infantile esotropia XLIV Edward Jackson memorial lecture. American Journal of Ophthalmology. 1988;**105**(1):1

[12] Schillinger RJ. A new type of tendon transplant operation for abducens paralysis. The Journal of the International College of Surgeons. 1959; **31**(5):593-600

[13] Phamonvaechavan P, Anwar D, Guyton DL. Adjustable suture technique for enhanced transposition surgery for extraocular muscles. Journal of American Association for Pediatric Ophthalmology and Strabismus. 2010; **14**(5):399-405

[14] Hummelsheim E. Weitere Erfahrungen mit partieller Sehnenuberpflanzung an den Augenmuskeln. Arch Augenheilkd. 1908;**62**:71-74

[15] Couser NL, Lenhart PD, Hutchinson AK. Augmented Hummelsheim procedure to treat complete abducens nerve palsy. Journal of American Association for Pediatric Ophthalmology and Strabismus. 2012; **16**(4):331-335

[16] Jensen CD. Rectus muscle union: A new operation for paralysis of the rectus muscle. Transactions of the Pacific Oto-Ophthalmological Society. 1964;**45**:359-387

[17] Nishida Y, Inatomi A, Aoki Y, Hayashi O, Iwami T, Oda S, et al. A muscle transposition procedure for abducens palsy, in which the halves of the vertical rectus muscle bellies are sutured onto the sclera. Japanese Journal of Ophthalmology. 2003;**47**(3):281-286

[18] Johnston SC et al. ARVO abstract. IOVS. 2006;**47**:2475:ARVO E-Abstract

[19] Velez FG, Chang MY, Pineles SL. Inferior rectus transposition: A novel procedure for abducens palsy. American Journal of Ophthalmology. 2017;**177**:126-130

[20] von Noorden GK. Anterior segment ischemia following the Jensen procedure. Archives of Ophthalmology. 1976;**94**(5):845-847

[21] Ruth AL, Velez FG, Rosenbaum AL. Management of vertical deviations after vertical rectus transposition surgery. Journal of American Association for Pediatric Ophthalmology and Strabismus. 2009;**13**(1):16-19

[22] Rush JA, Younge BR. Paralysis of cranial nerves III, IV, and VI: Cause and prognosis in 1,000 cases. Archives of Ophthalmology. 1981;**99**(1):76-79

[23] Kirkham TH. Inheritance of Duane's syndrome. The British Journal of Ophthalmology. 1970;**54**(5):323

[24] McKusick VA, O'Neill MJ. Duane Retraction Syndrome 1. Hereditary Ocular Disease. USA: University of Arizona, Department of Ophthalmology and Vision Science; 2016. Available from: http://disorders.eyes.arizona.edu/disorders/duane-retraction-syndrome-1 [Accessed: February 4, 2024]

[25] Elliot AJ. Duane's retraction syndrome. Proceedings of the Royal Society of Medicine. 1945;**XXXVIII**:463-465

[26] Barry BJ, Whitman MC, Hunter DG, et al. Duane Syndrome. 2007 May 25 [Updated 2019 Aug 29]. In: Adam MP, Feldman J, Mirzaa GM, et al., editors. GeneReviews® [Internet]. Seattle (WA): University of Washington, Seattle; 1993-2024. Available from: https://www.ncbi.nlm.nih.gov/books/NBK1190/ [Accessed: February 4, 2024]

[27] Murillo-Correa CE, Kon-Jara V, Engle EC, Zenteno JC. Clinical features associated with an I126M α2-chimaerin mutation in a family with autosomal-dominant Duane retraction syndrome. Journal of American Association for Pediatric Ophthalmology and Strabismus. 2009;**13**(3):245-248

[28] Miyake N, Andrews C, Fan W, He W, Chan WM, Engle EC. CHN1 mutations are not a common cause of sporadic Duane's retraction syndrome. American Journal of Medical Genetics. Part A. 2010;**152**(1):215

[29] Hotchkiss MG, Miller NR, Clark AW, Green WR. Bilateral Duane's retraction syndrome: A clinical-pathologic case report. Archives of Ophthalmology. 1980;**98**(5):870-874

[30] Duane TD. Clinical ophthalmology. In: Pediatric Ophthalmic Surgery. Vol. 6. Philadelphia, PA: Lippincott Williams & Wilkins; 1994

[31] Talebnejad MR, Sahraian N, Eghtedari M. Management of Duane's syndrome with botulinum toxin

injection. Iranian Journal of Ophthalmology. 2008;**20**(3):10-14

[32] Barbe ME, Scott WE, Kutschke PJ. A simplified approach to the treatment of Duane's syndrome. British Journal of Ophthalmology. 2004;**88**(1):131-138

[33] Duane TD. Clinical ophthalmology. In: Strabismus, Refraction, the Lens. Vol. 1. Philadelphia, PA: Lippincott Williams & Wilkins; 1993

[34] Jampolsky A. Duane syndrome. In: Rosenbaum AL, Santiago AP, editors. Clinical Strabismus Management. Philadelphia: W.B. Saunders & Co; 1999. p. 331

[35] Doyle JJ, Hunter DG. Transposition procedures in Duane retraction syndrome. Journal of American Association for Pediatric Ophthalmology and Strabismus. 2019;**23**(1):5-14

Chapter 4

Exodeviations: Etiology, Classification, Epidemiology, Risk Factors, Examination, Presentation and Treatment

Jelena Škunca Herman, Maja Malenica Ravlić, Lana Knežević and Blanka Doko Mandić

Abstract

In this chapter, we intend to present the disease entity, which will include definition, types of exodeviation, symptoms, etiology, risk factors and nonsurgical treatment, as well as surgical management. The types of exodeviations that will be included are pseudoexotropia, exophoria, intermittent exotropia, sensory exotropia, and consecutive exotropia. We will also write about diagnosis of the disease itself, which includes the basics of a strabological examination. There will be special attention paid to the intermittent exotropia considering that intermittent exotropia is the most common type of exodeviations, with a special focus on its treatment. Postoperative treatment options will also be topic to discuss.

Keywords: exophoria, intermittent exotropia, consecutive exotropia, exodeviation, exotropia treatment

1. Introduction

Exodeviations are horizontal deviations of the eye outward from the midline. In the field of strabismus research and treatment, there is no complete agreement regarding the etiology and classification of exodeviations. Exodeviations can vary in severity and can be constant or intermittent. Treatment options may include nonsurgical or surgical procedures depending on the underlying cause and the degree of misalignment. Asymptomatic patients and those with stable fusion mostly do not need treatment.

2. Etiology

The etiology of exodeviations, based on the theories put forth by Von Noorden [1], Duane [2] and Bielschowsky [3], is generally considered a combination of mechanical and innervational factors. Duane primarily proposed that exodeviations stem from an imbalance in the innervational control system that manages the active processes of convergence and divergence. He suggested that an exodeviation that is greater at a distance fixation than at near fixation is caused by hypertonicity of divergence. Conversely, a deviation that is greater at near fixation than at distance fixation is a result of convergence insufficiency. The balance between convergence and divergence plays a significant part, and their interplay may contribute to the exodeviation's characteristics.

Bielschowsky questioned Duane's theory, arguing that it did not consider the abnormal rest position associated with exodeviations. He further suggested some of these abnormal deviations could be influenced by anatomical and mechanical factors, such as the orbital shape and axis, interpupillary distance, the globe's size, and the extrabulbar tissues.

Von Noorden [1] and Burian [4] adds an innervational component to basic deviation caused by mechanical and anatomical factors, saying that the interplay between innervation influences that promote or impair ocular alignment is integral to the pathogenesis of exodeviations.

The modern understanding proposes that exodeviations are due to a combination of these theories, with mechanical and anatomical (static) factors contributing to a basic misalignment of the visual axes. This basic exotropia is affected by innervational (dynamic) factors that either maintain ocular alignment via convergence or impair it through divergence. Normal interplay between these forces will provide coarse alignment of the eyes, and any aberration in this is considered as a principal factor in the pathogenesis of exodeviations.

Refractive errors can also modify the innervational pattern that influences the eyes' position, a mechanism that underscores the role of myopia and hypermetropia in the etiology of exodeviations. Factors like anisomyopia and anisoastigmatism, which cause unequal retinal image clarity, could contribute to the pathogenesis of exotropia.

However, it is important to note that these theories and classifications of exodeviations were formulated descriptively, and there still exists a need for further understanding of its etiological intricacies.

3. Classification

Most of the current classifications for exodeviations trace back to Duane who proposed that exodeviations are a result of an innervational misproportion that disrupts the reciprocal relationship between active convergence and divergence mechanisms.

Considering the state of the vergence systems, we can use the concepts proposed by Duane once again (**Table 1**). These classifications do not bring about any direct etiological implications. But the angle of deviation can provide valuable insights into the nature of exodeviation. For instance, when the exodeviation at distance fixation is larger than that at near fixation, it suggests divergence excess. Conversely, if exodeviation is greater at near fixation than at distance fixation, the condition is indicative of convergence insufficiency. Basic exodeviation implies an angle that is equal at distance fixation and near fixation. Simulated divergence excess is the exodeviation that occurs when the disparity between distance and near deviations is not a fundamental characteristic of the exodeviation, but rather a temporary masking event influenced by persistent convergence innervation. Specific tests, such as the Scobee-Burian occlusion test that involves unilateral occlusion of one eye for a brief period (30–45 minutes), may be necessary to reveal the deviation at near fixation. Following such occlusion, it is often found that the near deviation equals or even exceeds the distance deviation [1].

The classification based on the state of fusion distinguishes between latent/manifest, intermittent, and constant exodeviation (**Table 1**) [1]:

Due to the state of vergence system	Due to the state of the fusion	Due to the typological terms
• Basic exodeviation	• Latent exodeviation	• Primary exotropia
• Divergence excess	• Exophoria	• Exophoria
• Convergence insufficiency	• Manifest exodeviation	• Intermittent exotropia
• Simulated divergence excess	• Intermittent exotropia	• Constant exotropia
	• Constant exotropia	• Secondary exotropia
		• Sensory
		• Consecutive

Table 1.
Classification of exotropia.

- Exophoria: Disorder occurs in states that interrupt fusion, when one eye is closed. This condition is typically detected during testing monocular visual acuity and performing an alternate cover test, when binocular vision is interrupted.

- Intermittent exotropia: It signifies a controlled form of exodeviation where the eyes are generally aligned but in relaxed or uncontrolled states (tiredness, daydreaming); one eye may drift outward. Intermittent exodeviation represents a disrupted state of fusion, occurring in periods when binocular vision is being used.

- Exotropia (constant exodeviation): This is identified when there's a constant loss of fusion and the eyes are constantly misaligned regardless of the distance of the fixation point.

On examining the state of fusion, the capacity of the patient to control exodeviation plays a crucial role. Patients with good control might be able to recover binocular fusion without any cue, but those with poor control might require visual cues such as a blink or refixation to regain binocular fusion.

Speaking in typological terms, exodeviations can be primary or secondary (**Table 1**).

- Primary exotropia (exophoria, intermittent exotropia, constant exotropia) typically has few or no identifiable secondary causes or associations. It is not linked to an underlying systemic condition or craniofacial anomaly, or is a result of ocular surgery, nor is it a consequence of sensory deficit. Essentially, primary exotropia arises independently, with no discernible etiological factors apart from possible innervational or mechanical elements. Types of primary exotropia often switch among each other [1].

- Secondary exotropia develops as a result of another condition or event. Unlike primary exotropia, this form of exotropia is not innate, but occurs due to underlying circumstances. It presents as a residual or secondary deviation following another condition and can arise either spontaneously in a formerly esotropic patient (one who had an inward turning of the eye) or iatrogenically after surgical overcorrection of an esodeviation. Two distinct forms of secondary exotropia include consecutive exotropia and sensory exotropia [1].

Due to the time of appearance	Due to the method of fixation
• Congenital or infantile	• Unilateral
• Acquired	• Alternating

Table 2.
Classification of exotropia.

According to the time of appearance: If the deviation is noted at birth or in the first months of life, it is considered congenital or infantile (**Table 2**). If it arises after that age, it is labeled as acquired.

With regard to the method of fixation, exodeviations can be either unilateral, with the patient habitually using one eye, or alternating, with the ability to fixate with either eye (**Table 2**). In alternating exotropia, either eye may deviate outward at different times, unlike constant or intermittent exotropia, which usually affects one eye.

The classification of exodeviations is vital when deciding the most suitable therapeutic approach for managing the condition, whether surgical or nonsurgical interventions are used. Moreover, the monitoring of exodeviations is critical as some exodeviations may progress or decompensate over time, making timely intervention necessary.

4. Epidemiology

Prevalence of exotropia can vary depending on the population sampled. In a meta-analysis study encompassing 56 articles by Hashemi et al. [5], the collected prevalence data suggests that exotropia occurs in approximately 1.23% of the population. This suggests that about 12 out of every 1000 individuals are affected by this condition.

If we look at specific manifestations of exotropia, the prevalence values can differ. For instance, a study conducted in China among preschool children revealed the prevalence of intermittent exotropia to be 3.24% [6]. In this particular population, nearly 33 out of 1000 individuals are impacted. This study did not observe any significant differences with regard to age (p-value = 0.19) or sex (p-value = 0.89). Additionally, among these patients, the most common form of intermittent exotropia was the "basic type", present in 74.7% of cases [6].

On the matter of incidence, Govindan et al. conducted a 10-year retrospective study in Minnesota that revealed an annual age- and gender-adjusted incidence of 64.1 per 100,000 patients aged 19 years or younger. In this study, the majority of cases, about 86% to be precise, were reported to involve intermittent exotropia or convergence insufficiency [7].

It is essential to remember that the prevalence and incidence of exotropia can vary based on geographical locations, populations sampled, and the type of exotropia being considered. As represented in the studies mentioned, while exotropia as a whole might be found at a lower rate in the general population, certain subtypes, such as intermittent exotropia, may present at higher rates within specific demographics.

5. Risk factors

Exotropia has several potential risk factors (**Table 3**). However, it is crucial to note that individual susceptibility to these factors can vary widely, and their presence does not assure the onset of the condition. Some risk factors for exotropia might include:

Risk factors
• smoking and substance abuse during pregnancy
• preterm birth and/or low birth weight
• age
• genetic factors
• ocular conditions (uncorrected refractive errors, sensory deprivation)
• neuromuscular abnormalities
• eye or orbital trauma
• systemic conditions (diabetes, thyroid disorders, cerebral palsy)

Table 3.
Risk factors for exotropia.

- Smoking and substance abuse during pregnancy
- Preterm birth and/or low birth weight
- Genetic factors: Familial history of any form of strabismus is a significant risk. If a parent or sibling has had either exotropia or esotropia, the risk increases.
- Ocular conditions:
  - Uncorrected refractive errors: High degrees of myopia, hyperopia, anisometropia, and amblyopia and impairment of binocular fusion (may be at a higher risk of developing exotropia, either due to the innate need for the eyes to compensate for these vision defects or due to complications from corrective surgeries)
  - Sensory deprivation: Vision loss in one eye (e.g., retinopathy of prematurity, corneal scars, cataracts, glaucoma, severe ptosis, and long-standing vitreous hemorrhage)
- Neuromuscular abnormalities: Abnormalities of the muscles that control the eye, or the nerves that stimulate those muscles, can lead to strabismus, including exotropia. Such problems can stem either from congenital conditions or from damage due to trauma, systemic disease, or degenerative conditions.
- Eye or orbital trauma: Injury to the structures surrounding the eye can impact the muscles that control eye movements and lead to strabismus.
- Systemic conditions: Certain systemic diseases like diabetes, thyroid disorders, cerebral palsy, and other neurologic impairment and craniofacial disorders can be associated with strabismus.
- Age: The onset of exotropia can occur at any age, but it most commonly begins either during early childhood or after the age of 50. Age can thus be seen as an influential factor in its occurrence.

These are general risk factors, and how they apply to individual patients will vary [8–12]. Medical consultation is recommended for the most accurate assessment of risk for any medical condition, including exotropia.

6. Clinical examination of exodeviation

The initial examination involves several steps, starting with a comprehensive history taking, followed by systematic visual examinations.

The very first step in a strabismus evaluation is the collection of a comprehensive and detailed history. Important topics to consider during this history-taking process include the nature of the symptoms the patient is experiencing, when these symptoms were first noticed, how they have changed over time, and any incidents of antecedent illnesses, trauma, surgeries, or blood loss that might be linked to the appearance of strabismus.

Following history-taking, the patient's current ophthalmic treatment regime is evaluated. The use of glasses or contact lenses, their prescription age, duration of use, and their effect on the strabismus are all documented. The use of prisms in their glasses or any history of occlusion therapy is likewise asked about.

The patient is then subjected to certain clinical examinations, divided into categories, which do not differ from other types of strabismus:

- Vision assessment: It incorporates standardized recognition distance and near visual acuity tests and orthoptic assessments, which include various tests such as the Hirschberg's and Bruckner's test and so on. These tests help to assess the vision and the binocular status of the patient.

- Assessment of binocular single vision (BSV): BSV should be evaluated through a stereopsis tests (e.g., Titmus test, Lang I, Lang II test), measuring the state of fusion and Bagolini's test for simultaneous perception. This assessment should be performed at every visit, and the results documented as the condition might worsen over time. Any significant progressive decline in stereopsis can serve as an early indicator for the need for surgical intervention.

- Ocular motility examination: It requires the patient to gaze in nine diagnostic positions (straight ahead, left, right, up, down, upper/left right, lower/left right). The scope of each eye's movements in each direction is observed to identify abnormalities such as limited movements or irregular eye rotations.

- Binocular alignment: Evaluated with a cover/uncover test and alternate cover test. The goal is to identify whether a tropia or deviation in eye alignment exists.

- Angle of deviation: It is measured at near and distance with Prism Cover test and Alternate Prism Cover test.

- Physical examination: The conditions of the eyelids, lacrimal drainage system, the conjunctiva, the cornea, and other ocular structures are carefully examined.

In certain cases, additional techniques and more specialized tests such as Maddox rod testing, Tangent Screen, Bielschowsky's test, fundus photography, and Hess screen testing may be utilized to evaluate ocular alignment or to measure cyclotropia. Other examinations may include an ocular muscle light reflex test, a red glass test, and an ocular deviation measurement using different devices.

It is worth noting the information obtained from these tests will influence the decision-making process in the management and treatment of the strabismus.

The process of clinical examination specific for exodeviation involves several strategies and tests:

- Fusional amplitudes: Patient's convergence and divergence amplitudes should also be measured. Most patients with intermittent exotropia have adequate convergence amplitudes for near but poor-to-adequate amplitudes for distance. Divergence amplitudes in these patients are usually normal.

- Occlusion test (Scobee-Burian): This test removes the vergence aftereffect, and it is crucial for distinguishing true from simulated divergence excess. Test becomes critical when a patient present with symptoms such as an intermittent exotropia that is present only at a distance, or a deviation at a distance exceeding the near deviation by 15 prism diopters (PD) or more. In the occlusion test, one eye is occluded for a minimum of 45 minutes, and then, the squint measurements are repeated using the alternate prism cover test. Any pronounced increase in the post-occlusion near angle of deviation can be labeled as simulated divergence excess exotropia. Should the near deviation remain the same, this condition is classified as true divergence excess exotropia.

- +3 diopter spherical lens test: This test removes accommodation and accommodative convergence, and it is important in detecting exotropia with high accommodative convergence/accommodation (AC/A) ratio. In this test, the exodeviations for near are measured with and without a +3 diopter spherical lens placed in front of the exotropic eye while using an accommodative target. This method helps estimate the AC/A ratio. The near angle of deviation in exotropia with a low AC/A ratio will increase minimum when +3 diopter spherical lens test is placed, but in exotropia with a high AC/A ratio, it will increase significantly [1].

7. Clinical presentation

Exodeviations encompass a group of ocular conditions wherein a visible deviation of the eye is observed, in an outward direction relative to the straight or forward gaze (**Figure 1**). The forms of exodeviations include exophoria, intermittent exotropia, (constant) exotropia, and sensory and consecutive exotropia. These ocular deviations can exhibit distinctive symptoms and complications and are an integral part of strabismus disorders. In this chapter, it is also important to mention pseudostrabismus, a false strabismus.

7.1 Pseudostrabismus

Pseudostrabismus is a term used to describe the appearance of strabismus even though the eyes are properly aligned. This is often due to certain facial features, such as a wide nasal bridge, prominent epicanthal folds (a fold of skin that comes down across the inner angle of the eye), or close-set eyes, all of which can make it appear

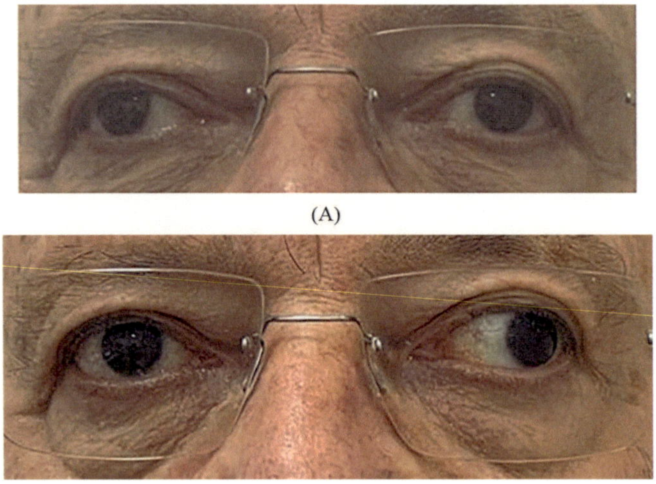

(A)

(B)

Figure 1.
Alternating exodeviation; exodeviation of right eye (A), and exodeviation of the left eye (B).

as though the eyes are turning outward or inward. In pseudostrabismus, the eye alignment is normal and binocular vision is intact. Over time, as the child's facial features mature and change, the appearance of eye misalignment often disappears. It is essential to differentiate between pseudostrabismus and true strabismus, since the latter requires treatment to prevent long-term visual impairment.

The differentiation between pseudostrabismus and strabismus can be made using a combination of detailed history taking, visual examination, and diagnostic tests.

To distinguish between pseudostrabismus and true strabismus, a basic examination would involve the observation of corneal light reflexes (Hirschberg test). In true strabismus, the corneal reflex will be off-center in the deviating eye. In pseudostrabismus, despite the appearance, the corneal reflex will be central in both eyes, indicating that the eyes are indeed aligned. There are circumstances when the eyes are aligned but the corneal reflex is displaced from the center for which the kappa angle is responsible. Angle kappa refers to the vergence of the visual axis from the pupillary axis, which is triggered by the anatomical arrangement where the fovea is slightly displaced from the optic axis. A positive angle kappa, which means the corneal light reflex is displaced nasalward, may simulate a pseudoexotropia. This can also make an existing exodeviation look worse than it actually is, or it may even mask or conceal an entire or part of an esodeviation.

The most common cause of pseudoexotropia is retinopathy of prematurity, while other causes include vascular abnormalities, macular scars, choroiditis, and other peripheral retinal disorders that cause traction (e.g., familial exudative vitreoretinopathy, toxocara retinitis, incontinentia pigmenti) [13] and orbital deformities or tumors that cause dystropia but not true strabismus. Pseudoexotropia can also occur in children with temporal dragging of the macula secondary to retinal traction.

Pseudoexotropia can be differentiated from true strabismus with the cover/uncover test and alternate test. In pseudostrabismus, no movement should be visible when either eye is covered.

If there should be any degree of unreliability in the diagnosis of pseudostrabismus, a complete eye examination may be warranted. There should certainly be regular checkups to ensure normal visual development and promptly identify any potential ocular issues.

In summary, pseudostrabismus, while giving the appearance of eye misalignment, does not entail the actual eye misalignment or binocular vision disruption seen in actual strabismus. It is a facet of an individual's physical appearance that typically resolves with growth and maturation and does not typically necessitate treatment.

7.2 Exophoria

Exophoria is a type of latent deviation where the eyes tend to deviate outward, but it is only detectable under particular viewing conditions. Typically, it is observed when binocular vision is interrupted, such as during an alternate cover test or monocular visual acuity testing. This condition is usually asymptomatic. However, patients with exophoria may experience asthenopia, or eye strain, with prolonged near work. Decompensation of an exophoria to an exotropia can occur under certain situations such as when the patient is ill or under the influence of alcohol or sedatives. When exophoria decompensated, diplopia appears. During the regular examination, a rapid change from phoria to tropia can also be observed. This is possible due to fusional amplitude control, relationship between convergence and accommodation, and variable deviation angle at different fixation difference [1]. Treatment is generally recommended when the exophoria becomes symptomatic.

7.3 Exotropia

Exotropia, on the other hand, is a more severe form of exodeviation that is more readily apparent and often manifests even under normal binocular viewing conditions. It is characterized by a manifest and more consistent outward turning of one or both eyes. But from time to time, it is difficult to distinguish between exophoria and exotropia. The exodeviation becomes manifest during times of visual inattention, fatigue, stress, or illness. It is often accompanied by symptoms such as visual disruption and decreased stereopsis (depth perception), and in adults, it can lead to significant psychological stress, anxiety, and depression. Primary exotropia is further divided into intermittent and constant exotropia. Small angle exotropia is generally rare, and the angle is mainly greater than 20 PD.

7.3.1 Intermittent exotropia

The most common type of exotropia and the most common exodeviation of childhood is intermittent exotropia, affecting approximately 1% of the general population [14]. It typically occurs at the age of 2–3 years [15] and often continues into adulthood.

It is an intermittent ocular condition, meaning it appears and disappears over time, often influenced by the focusing attention of the individual. Distance fixation may frequently induce the manifestation of an exotropic shift. On the other hand, near fixation, or focusing on objects close to the eyes, generally results in a normal binocular alignment, signifying that bifoveal fixation can be achieved in such cases. Clinically, symptoms of intermittent exotropia may include squinting or closing one eye when exposed to bright light, eye strain, or complaints of blurred vision. They help reestablish fusion by blinking, which may be one of the presenting complaint [16]. There is also the visual symptom of manifest exotropia, particularly when the individual is inattentive, fatigued, or focusing on distant objects. However, typically, intermittent exotropia does not have diplopia, and the vision remains unaffected, except in cases when the condition progress into a constant form of exotropia. In certain cases, intermittent exotropia may also convert into other types of strabismus. The control of the manifest exodeviation can lessen over time, expanding to both near and distant fixation, in addition to happening more frequently or continuously. Children with intermittent exotropia have less risk of developing amblyopia than those with esotropia.

Intermittent exotropia can be categorized according to the angle of exodeviation and AC/A ratio [17]:

- Basic exotropia is an exodeviation that is approximately the same size at distance and at near fixation

- Convergence insufficiency exotropia is exodeviation that is greater at near compared with at distance fixation. The angle of deviation is at least 10 PD larger at near than at distance. It may be associated with asthenopia or diplopia with reading and near work.

- Divergence excess exotropia is exodeviation that is greater at distance compared with at near fixation. The angle of deviation is at least 10–15 PD larger at distance than at near. As we mentioned earlier, it is important to distinguish true from simulated divergence excess with occlusion test. If there is a difference in the angle of deviation even after occlusion, the true divergence excess is present. The next step is to do a +3 diopter spherical lens test to differentiate low/normal from high AC/A ratio.

- Exotropia with high (AC/A) ratio. The AC/A ratio refers to the relationship between the accommodative convergence (the inward turning of the eyes that occurs when one attempts to see a close object clearly) and the accommodation (the adjustment of the lens of the eye for near vision). A high AC/A ratio indicates that a relatively large amount of convergence is associated with a unit of accommodation. Therefore, exotropia with a high AC/A ratio gives the appearance of a divergent excess and a smaller angle of deviation at near, which will increase and may equal to that at distance after the +3 diopter spherical lens test is performed.

7.3.2 Constant exotropia

Constant exotropia is a condition where the patient is consistently unable to align both eyes on a single object, resulting in a persistent outward deviation of the eye. This is often present in the elderly with long-standing intermittent exotropia that has decompensated or those with sensory, infantile, and consecutive exotropia. The same forms can be observed as in intermittent exotropia. Patients with constant exotropia may have an increased field of peripheral vision and may experience a constriction of their field of vision when their eyes are realigned.

7.4 Sensory exotropia

Sensory exotropia may develop due to visual deprivation in one eye that significantly disrupt or completely destroy the fusion mechanism, resulting in strabismus. This can be the result of a range of pathologic conditions that reduce visual acuity in one eye, including anisometropia, injuries, corneal opacities, congenital or traumatic unilateral cataracts, congenital glaucoma, macular lesions, optic atrophy, and vitreous hemorrhage [1]. The deviation is unilateral, with the amblyopic eye being the one typically affected. In general, when the onset of visual impairment occurs at birth or between birth and 5 years of age, both sensory esotropia and exotropia occur with almost equal frequency. After 5 years of age, sensory exotropia predominates. However, the mechanism leading to exotropia in some patients and esotropia in others with visual impairment remains unclear.

The presence of sensory exotropia suggests an absence of normal binocular function due to the visual disparity between the two eyes. With sensory exotropia, neither normal retinal correspondence (which occurs in normal binocular vision, where similar points on each retina correspond and present a single visual field to the brain) nor anomalous retinal correspondence (a variant of normal binocular vision, often seen in strabismus, where non-corresponding points on each retina provide a single visual field to the brain) is at play. Over time, suppression can become more deeply established, reinforcing the use of only one eye for sight and reducing the chances of establishing or reestablishing BSV.

7.5 Consecutive exotropia

Consecutive exotropia arises as a result of undergoing surgery for the correction of esotropia, which is much more common, or as a spontaneous shift from esotropia to exotropia [1].

There are multiple factors that may contribute to the onset of consecutive exotropia. For postsurgical cases, it may occur due to an overcorrection of the initial esodeviation during the surgical intervention. When consecutive exotropia arises spontaneously, it may be associated with poor vision in the deviating eye, as seen in sensory exotropia. However, not all cases can be explained on this basis alone. High hypermetropia in an esotropic patient may be another contributing factor, as a shift to consecutive exotropia is frequently observed in this group of patients.

8. Treatment

The treatment approach for exodeviations typically depends on the patient's specific condition and can encompass a variety of strategies aiming to improve visual alignment and normal binocular function. The approach may vary from noninvasive measures such as spectacle correction, orthoptics, and occlusion therapy to surgical intervention. The treatment for congenital exotropia begins with amblyopia therapy. It is generally surgical for symptomatic exophoria, intermittent, and constant exotropia [1].

8.1 Nonsurgical treatment

Certain nonsurgical options may be considered to create optimal sensory conditions by stimulating fusion and maintaining active accommodative convergence before surgery or when surgery must be postponed [1]:

- Spectacle (contact lenses) prescription:
  - Correction of the refractive error (astigmatismus, anisometropia, myopia, hypermetropia): It is a first-line treatment. This process can better the retinal image's clarity, which increases the stimulus to fuse and aids control of the exodeviation. Full correction of myopia is required to preserve active accommodative convergence. The correction of any hypermetropic refractive error could decrease the demand on accommodative convergence and thus increase the exodeviation. Therefore, individual patient evaluations need to consider the degree of hypermetropia, patient age, and the AC/A ratio. Typically, in children with exodeviations, a hypermetropia of less than 2.00 Dsph is not routinely corrected. Hypermetropia correction in elderly is mandatory to avoid asthenopia. As a result of a correction, exophoria may worsen and may require treatment [1].
  - Overcorrecting minus lens therapy/over minus correction: This involves the prescription of myopic spectacles, commonly referred to as over-minus lenses. In some instances, overcorrection of myopia may stimulate accommodative convergence, thereby helping manage the exodeviation.
  - Treatment with prisms: The basic principle for prescribing prismatic correction is the elimination of asthenopic symptoms and the restoration of binocular vision. The indication for prescribing prisms is exophoria and manifest strabismus $\leq$10 PD with the potential of binocularity [18]. Although some strabologists prescribe prisms preoperatively to improve fusional control and bifoveal stimulation [19–21], Von Noorden [1] do not use prisms preoperatively. Some prescribe prisms postoperatively in patients with a small residual angle of deviation.
- Orthoptics (vision therapy):
  - Passive vision therapy/eye patching for amblyopia treatment is strongly recommended.
  - Active vision therapy/orthoptic exercises (combination of eye exercises and vision-training): The efficiency of orthoptic exercises in the treatment of exodeviations is doubtful. According to critical evaluation of the behavioural vision therapy and systematic review of the efficacy of eye exercises, there was no clear evidence-based studies to support these training and their use remains controversial [22, 23]. Although there is some evidence-based studies that support orthoptic exercises in the treatment of convergence insufficiency according to Arnoldi's review of convergence insufficiency, convergence exercises are only temporarily effective in improving proximal and tonic convergence, but the effect on fusional and accommodative convergence is little [24]. Sensory training to treat binocular vision anomalies should not be used as a substitute for surgery!

However, recent investigations have suggested that evidence regarding the efficacy of nonsurgical managements of exodeviations is still somewhat inconclusive, with the need for more comprehensive randomized controlled trial studies.

DOI: http://dx.doi.org/10.5772/intechopen.1002758

8.2 Surgical treatment

Surgical intervention is usually considered when nonsurgical options do not alleviate the condition. The need for surgery depends on the state of fusional control, the angle size of deviation, and patient age. Surgery in exotropia patients can be challenging, and postoperative care and recovery could require additional supporting measures. A crucial one to note is that strabismus surgery is not cosmetic; it is reconstructive. But in some cases, it can be just cosmetic (e.g., sensory exotropia, constant exotropia).

A key consideration before opting for surgical treatment is the regular monitoring of the patient. Signs indicative of the necessity for surgery include steady deterioration of fusional control, increased frequency of the manifest phase of the strabismus, or development of suppression. Functionally, if the exotropia presents more than 50% of waking hours or induces asthenopic problems, surgery is necessary [1].

The surgical treatment of exodeviations involves several careful steps to ensure a successful outcome and restoration of BSV. When planning the procedure, the surgeon must consider the severity of the condition, the obstruction of vision, the patient's age, and any underlying health conditions.

A step-by-step guide to the surgical treatment of exodeviations:

- Preoperative preparation: Before surgery, it is necessary to provide optimal sensory conditions as described earlier.

- Surgical planning: The surgeon evaluates the type and degree of exodeviation in order to plan the appropriate surgical approach. This planning involves considerations on whether unilateral or bilateral surgery is required.

- Prism adaptation test (PAT): it is used before every surgery, and it serves as a valuable diagnostic tool utilized to determine the "maximum" angle of squint before proceeding with eye muscle surgery. The primary objective of this assessment is to identify the extent of squint that can be effectively corrected while achieving the most optimal binocular outcome. The ultimate goal is to ensure accurate correction and avoid the possibility of undercorrection, thus enhancing the success of the surgical intervention.

- Anesthesia: Patients undergoing exodeviation surgery are typically given a general or local anesthesia, depending on their age and health conditions. The objective is to ensure they remain comfortable and pain-free during the procedure.

- Surgery: In the surgery, the surgeon alters the balance of the muscles by either strengthening the inward-pulling muscles, weakening the outward-pulling muscles, or a combination of both. In most cases, a resection (to strengthen a muscle) or recession (to weaken a muscle) procedure is performed. The eye muscles are carefully detached from their original position on the eye, repositioned, and reattached in a calculated location to adjust the pull of the muscles for better alignment.

- Closure: Once the muscles have been adjusted, the surgeon uses absorbable sutures to close the conjunctiva. Antibiotic eye ointments are applied to prevent infection.

- Immediate postoperative care: After the surgery, patients might occasionally experience double vision in the immediate postoperative period. Surgeons may prescribe short-term topical steroids and antibiotics, along with oral analgetics on a case-by-case basis for pain management and to prevent inflammation and infection.

- Follow-up visits: The postoperative care in patients who undergo surgical intervention should focus on alignment and correction of any underlying refractive errors. If necessary, prisms or occlusion glasses are advised if diplopia persists.

- Ongoing monitoring: Patients should continue to have regular follow-up appointments with their ophthalmologist to monitor the success of the surgery.

Consequently, the treatment administered is multifaceted, taking into account the patient's age, the severity and frequency of the strabismus, the control of the deviation, and the response to initial treatment methods. Thus, the approach is generally individualized to obtain optimal outcomes.

8.3 Exophoria

Asymptomatic patients with exophoria without muscular asthenopia typically do not require treatment. In contrast, symptomatic exophoria is typically approached with a surgical treatment strategy. But there are some situations in which the first attempt is to treat exophoria conservatively.

Nonsurgical treatment

- Spectacle (contact lenses) prescription:
    - Correction of the refractive error as mentioned earlier.
    - Bifocal lenses (the weakest) are prescribed in symptomatic exophoric patient with presbyopia before estimating the increase in exodeviation [1].
    - Treatment with prisms: If treatment with the weakest bifocals fails and patient still has symptoms, it is recommended to prescribe prisms base-in for near vision. Only about half of the angle is corrected with prisms. This is how accommodative convergence is stimulated [1].

Surgical treatment

- A more detailed description is in the chapter Treatment/exotropia/intermittent exotropia.

8.4 Exotropia

The management of exotropia depends on the type of exodeviation and any associated ocular findings. The standard surgical interventions for exophoria or exotropia include the recession of the lateral rectus muscle and resection of the medial rectus muscle. Surgeries can be performed unilaterally or bilaterally, depending on the individual patient's condition and the surgeon's judgment. Surgical treatment for exophoria and exotropia is typically directed at restoring optimal sensory conditions and at normalizing binocular function. The less experienced ophthalmologist might view the treatment of this condition with optimism, particularly given that a substantial number of patients demonstrate potential for reconstructing fusion and improvement in distance stereoacuity following surgery. But basically, the treatment is demanding and frustrating due to temporary improvement and frequent relapses. Postoperative care is crucial for ensuring the effectiveness of the surgical intervention. This includes focusing on eye alignment, managing any blinding complications, and correcting underlying refractive errors.

8.4.1 Intermittent exotropia

The treatment for intermittent exotropia can involve both surgical and nonsurgical options depending on the case's severity and specifics. The management strategies for intermittent exotropia can vary, but the main goals are to correct the eye misalignment, restore binocular vision, and prevent amblyopia. However, treating exotropia, whether intermittent or constant, can be a complex and intricate process.

Nonsurgical treatment

- Observation: In cases where patients are asymptomatic, intermittent exotropia is mild, has good control, and is not increasing; observation may be sufficient, as noted by Hutchinson [14]. The prognosis for normal binocular vision and stereopsis is good if the intermittent exotropia is rarely manifested. This approach entails diligent monitoring for associated issues such as amblyopia, eye strain, diplopia, closing of one eye in sunlight (monocular manifest deviation), increased frequency of deviation, and headaches. Decisions on intervention for children with intermittent exotropia should be made on a case-by-case basis by healthcare professionals and parents.

- Spectacle (contact lenses) prescription:

    - Correction of the refractive error as mentioned earlier.

    - Overcorrecting minus lens therapy/over minus correction: Von Noorden use this treatment only as a temporary measure in patients with a high AC/A ratio [1]. The rationale behind this approach was the anticipation that over-minus lenses could potentially enhance the management of intermittent exotropia by inducing accommodation and accommodative convergence. Despite this initial hypothesis, the findings of a 12-month randomized trial conducted on children aged 3–10 years yielded contrasting results. The trial revealed that while over-minus spectacles did indeed contribute to improved control of distance exotropia while the over-minus spectacles were worn, the beneficial effect did not persist after the treatment regimen was gradually tapered off. Additionally, an association was observed between the use of over-minus lenses and an increased myopic shift in participants [25]. Consequently, based on these outcomes, it is recommended to refrain from prescribing over-minus lenses for the specific purpose of managing intermittent exotropia. This suggestion is informed by the trial's results and the potential for unintended myopic progression associated with their usage.

- Treatment with prisms: The only indication for prescribing base-in prisms in exotropia is exotropia with small angle (≤10 PD) and with the potential of binocularity, as we mentioned earlier [18]. However, the use of base-in prisms for long-term management is not ideal as they can reduce fusional vergence amplitudes.

- Orthoptics (vision therapy):

  - Passive vision therapy/eye patching involves alternating part-time occlusion of one eye to counteract or diminish suppression. A randomized trial involving 201 young children with intermittent exotropia compared part-time patching to observation, revealing uncommon deterioration over 6 months in both groups (2.2% versus 4.6%, respectively; nonsignificant) [26]. Although exotropia control was slightly better with patching (mean score 2.3 versus 2.8), this distinction may lack clinical significance. A similar study in older children (ages 3 to <11 years), also from PEDIG group, indicated that part-time patching reduced deterioration over 6 months, with infrequent deterioration in both groups (0.6% in patching versus 6.1% in observation) [27]. As with other treatments for intermittent exotropia, therapy discontinuation often results in failure and recurrence [28]. Von Noorden [1] occasionally found it useful using alternating occlusion instead of surgery in patients with small-angle intermittent exotropia.

  - Active vision therapy/orthoptic exercises enhance convergence/divergence amplitudes, fusion strength, and single binocular vision [29]. Typically administered by experienced optometrists, this treatment often involves office-based sessions supplemented by at-home exercises. Alternatively, it can be entirely conducted at home through computer-generated orthoptic exercises. In a randomized controlled trial of 221 children (ages 9–17 years), an intensive program of office-based vision therapy with home reinforcement proved more effective in reducing signs and symptoms compared to various home-based therapies [30]. "Active" vision therapy entailed a comprehensive protocol incorporating diverse exercises targeting improved vergence and accommodation. Conversely, the control intervention consisted of home-based procedures simulating orthoptic exercises without vergence or accommodation training. While this study suggests the superiority of intensive office-based vision therapy over home-based therapy devoid of binocular vision training, further research is warranted to ascertain if office-based therapy surpasses equally intensive home-based therapy [31]. Despite the fact that some countries and some strabologists implement active vision therapy, as mentioned earlier, evidence-based studies are lacking and their effectiveness is questionable [31].

Surgical treatment

Intermittent exotropia may not always require immediate surgery. Taking into account that it does not progress in all patients, patients must be observed for several months. Surgery is typically recommended when certain signs or symptoms are present in the patient, or they develop while the patient is under monitored observation. These may include gradual loss of fusional control demonstrated by increasing frequency of the manifest phase of the strabismus, development of secondary convergence insufficiency, increase in size of the basic deviation, development of suppression evidenced by absence of diplopia during the manifest phase of the strabismus, or a decrease of stereoacuity. In simpler terms, when the exotropia happens more than 50% of the patient's waking hours or causes asthenopic problems, surgery is advised [1]. Despite this, it is important to note that surgical treatment of intermittent exotropia or constant exotropia, especially after a long period of intermittency, is generally aimed at normalization of binocular function.

The ideal age at which surgery should be performed has been a subject of debate. Some experts argue that surgery in visually immature infants should be delayed to avoid consecutive esotropia. On the other hand, others argue in favor of early surgical intervention. According to Baker et al. [32] and Von Noorden [1], surgery for intermittent exotropia should be postponed until the fourth year of life. Earlier surgical intervention is usually recommended if there is a rapid functional deterioration of fusional control despite nonsurgical therapy or if the deviation is constant. Despite the fact that the minimum preoperative angle of deviation should not be less than 15 PD, the angle of deviation greater than 20/25 PD is mostly operated [1]. In conclusion, strabismus surgery stands as the predominant treatment for advanced intermittent exotropia, or when nonsurgical methods prove insufficient [33]. Surgical guidelines advocate intervention for frequent exodeviation manifestation and symptomatic patients. Those conditions in which the patient is asymptomatic with stable fusion at distance and near are considered to be cured [1].

The preferred surgical treatment for intermittent exotropia (and exophoria), varies with the specific attributes of the deviation, including the size and nature of the deviation, the presence or absence of near-distance disparity, and the surgeon's preference. However, some common surgical interventions include:

- Two-muscle unilateral surgery (asymmetrical surgery): In this procedure, the medial rectus muscle of one eye is resected, and the lateral rectus muscle of the same eye is recessed (**Figure 2**). This aims to adjust the balance of forces acting on the eye and realign the visual axis.

- Bilateral surgery (symmetrical surgery): In this approach, the lateral rectus muscle is recessed in both eyes. Resection of the medial muscles can also be done.

- One-muscle unilateral surgery: In some cases, only one lateral rectus muscle will be recessed. This procedure may be advisable for small-angle deviations or in situations where the risk of overcorrection might be particularly concerning.

The choice of surgical method depends on several factors. It is crucial to distinguish true from the simulated divergence excess. According to Burian, when there is a true divergence excess, bilateral lateral rectus recession might be the preferred choice. Two-muscle unilateral surgery (recession of the lateral rectus muscle with resection of the ipsilateral medial rectus muscle) on the nondominant eye is the procedure of choice for basic exotropia or the simulated divergence excess [34–36]. Other authors showed the same effectiveness of bilateral recession of the lateral rectus muscles in case of basic exotropia and in case of simulated divergent excess [37]. Conversely, for near exotropias (convergence insufficiency), both medial rectus resection from 3 to 6 mm might be utilized [1, 38]. However, there are cases where a surgeon chooses to perform a recess-resect procedure for all types of exotropia. When asymmetric surgery is the method of choice, then the nondominant eye is operated on.

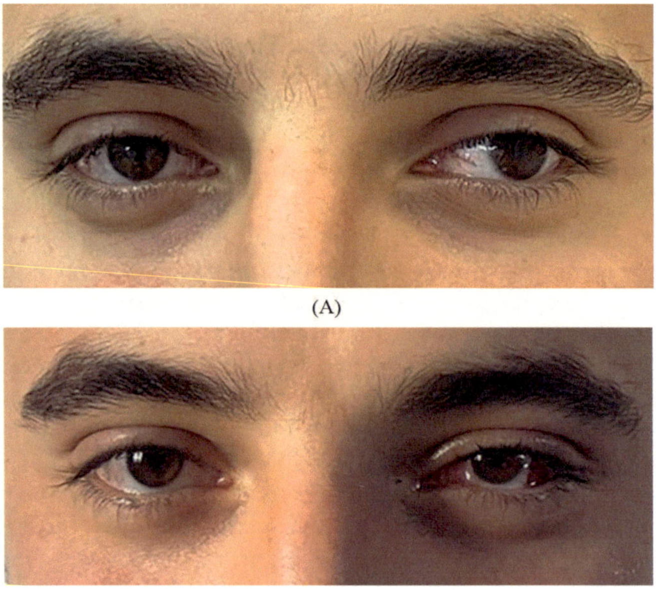

(A)

(B)

Figure 2.
Left eye exotropia before surgery (A) and first postoperative day after two-muscle unilateral surgery (B).

A variety of treatments have been proposed for intermittent exotropia; however, there is no universally superior approach for all cases. Studies have shown no statistically significant differences in outcomes between these surgical strategies. Some showed better early postoperative effect with asymmetrical surgery [39]. Long-term follow-up demonstrates a high recurrence rate regardless of the initial therapy chosen [28, 40, 41]. Additionally, the evolving landscape of medical knowledge and practice may provide further insights into refining these treatment strategies. A key objective in this line of treatment is to relieve symptoms, reduce the frequency of manifest deviation, decrease the angle of deviation, and enhance the individual's control over it.

It was also suggested that an initial overcorrection of around 10–20 PD in the immediate postoperative period might be advantageous in terms of long-term outcomes. It is considered as an attempt to extend the effect of the surgical procedure. Less than that causes relapse, and more than 10–20 PD causes consecutive esotropia [1]. Though, it is noted that consecutive esotropia frequently recovers over time, there is no consensus about this, as overcorrection could even provoke diplopia. In general, the response to these different treatment strategies is variable, and more randomized controlled trial studies are needed to conclusively establish the most effective approach.

8.4.2 Constant exotropia

In case of constant exotropia, preoperative nonsurgical treatment is not required. If constant exotropia occurs in early infancy and if there is no data on intermittency, the functional prognosis is poor. Surgery should be performed as soon as the angle of deviation can be measured, which must be at least 15 PD, and when the child alternates freely. Mostly, it is between the first and second year of life. Adults are operated on as soon as the diagnosis is confirmed. Unfortunately, in such cases, the establishment of BSV is not expected [1].

Surgical treatment for constant exotropia is similar to that for intermittent exotropia. However, one notable aspect is that recurrence rates are high, as shown in long-term follow-up studies for the surgical treatment of intermittent exotropia. Therefore, patients may require multiple surgeries to maintain ocular alignment over a long period. Furthermore, it is worth noting that some consider a delay in surgical treatment as a risk factor for the recurrence of strabismus.

8.5 Sensory exotropia

The management goal in sensory exotropia focuses less on restoring binocular visual function and more on alleviating the noticeable eye divergence for aesthetic and comfort purposes. Surgical procedure is the same as that for intermittent exotropia.

8.6 Consecutive exotropia

The specific procedure to correct consecutive exotropia largely depends on individual patient conditions. Consecutive exotropia that arises spontaneously generally requires a surgical intervention to restore normal facial configuration. The goal of the surgery is to realign the eyes to improve cosmetic appearance and potentially visual function. The indications for this surgery are often cosmetic. The most widely used surgical procedures for consecutive exotropia are the same as those for other types of exotropia. However, the exact method may vary based on the specific characteristics of the patient's strabismus. Postoperatively, the patients regularly have follow-up visits to assess their eye alignment, ocular motility, correction of underlying refractive errors, and the possible development of postoperative diplopia.

It is crucial to note that postoperative management and prognosis will vary depending on the specifics of each case, including the extent of the exotropia, the patient's age, and other individual health factors. Therefore, a personalized treatment and postoperative management plan is essential for each case.

8.7 Postsurgical treatment of undercorrections

After exodeviation surgery, in some patients, the residual deviation is visible immediately after the operation and will require additional surgery, while in others, it occurs only a few months or even years after the initially satisfactory result. In such cases, the use of base-in prisms with a power base greater than the residual deviation is recommended to promote convergence and restore fusion amplitudes with the goal of reducing exodeviation [1]. Unfortunately, additional surgery is required in most cases.

8.8 Postsurgical treatment of overcorrections (consecutive exotropia)

According to different authors, the prevalence of surgical overcorrections in patients with exodeviations varies from 6% to 20% [35, 36, 42–45]. Observation is the therapy of choice for minor degrees of esotropia, which are usually comitant in nature. Postoperative esodeviation of 10–15 PD is desirable and may disappear completely over time, but larger deviations tend to increase. In the first 6 months postoperatively, no other surgery should be performed except when there are significant duction limitations causing an unrelated lateral view.

During observation, several nonsurgical treatment methods can be performed to reduce postoperative deviation or, if this is not possible, to maintain fusion and ensure patient comfort. When diplopia persists for 2 weeks after surgery, miotics or a temporary prescription for hyperopic refractive error can reduce the deviation to the point where the patient will converge. If this therapy is inefficacious, diplopia can be eliminated with alternating occlusion, which will also tend to reduce the angle of successive esotropia. Base outward prisms are a common treatment option, especially when fusion must be maintained under all circumstances, such as in visually immature children or for professional reasons in adults [44, 46]. Many difficulties of this form of therapy that were previously encountered have been eliminated by the use of press-on Fresnel membrane. In the treatment of patients with retained motor fusion, injections of botulinum toxin into the medial rectus muscle have also been shown to be beneficial [47].

The treatment of permanent consecutive esotropia requires considerable patience of the doctor, because the spontaneous reduction of the postoperative angle may take a long time. According to Hardesty and his coworkers [42], consecutive esotropia of less than 15 can be cured with prism therapy alone, whereas surgery usually becomes necessary for larger esodeviations.

Conflict of interest

The authors declare no conflict of interest.

Author details

Jelena Škunca Herman*, Maja Malenica Ravlić, Lana Knežević
and Blanka Doko Mandić
Department of Ophthalmology, University Hospital Centre Sestre Milosrdnice,
Zagreb, Croatia

*Address all correspondence to: jskuncaherman@gmail.com

References

[1] Von Noorden GK. Exodeviations. In: von Noorden GK, Campos EC, editors. Binocular Vision and Ocular Motility: Theory and Management of Strabismus. 6th ed. St. Louis, Missouri: Mosby Inc; 2002. pp. 356-376

[2] Duane A. A new classification of the motor anomalies of the eyes based upon physiological principles, together with their symptoms, diagnosis and treatment. Annals of Ophthalmology and Otology. 1897;**6**:84,247

[3] Bielschowsky A. Divergence excess. Archives of Ophthalmology. 1934;**12**(2):157-166. DOI: 10.1001/archopht.1934.00830150011001

[4] Burian HM. Pathophysiology of exodeviations. In: Manley DR, editor. Symposium on Horizontal Ocular Deviations. St Louis: Mosby Inc; 1971. p. 119

[5] Hashemi H, Pakzad R, Heydarian S, Yekta A, Aghamirsalim M, Shokrollahzadeh F, et al. Global and regional prevalence of strabismus: a comprehensive systematic review and meta-analysis. Strabismus. 2019;**27**(2):54-65. DOI: 10.1080/09273972.2019.1604773

[6] Pan CW, Zhu H, Yu JJ, Ding H, Bai J, Chen J, et al. Epidemiology of intermittent exotropia in preschool children in China. Optometry and Vision Science. 2016;**93**(1):57-62. DOI: 10.1097/OPX.0000000000000754

[7] Govindan M, Mohney BG, Diehl NN, Burke JP. Incidence and types of childhood exotropia: a population-based study. Ophthalmology. 2005;**112**(1):104-108. DOI: 10.1016/j.ophtha.2004.07.033

[8] O'Connor AR, Stephenson TJ, Johnson A, et al. Strabismus in children of birth weight less than 1701 g. Archives of Ophthalmology. 2002;**120**:767. DOI: 10.1001/archopht.120.6.767

[9] Holmström G, el Azazi M, Kugelberg U. Ophthalmological follow up of preterm infants: a population based, prospective study of visual acuity and strabismus. The British Journal of Ophthalmology. 1999;**83**:143. DOI: 10.1136/bjo.83.2.143

[10] Pennefather PM, Clarke MP, Strong NP, et al. Risk factors for strabismus in children born before 32 weeks' gestation. The British Journal of Ophthalmology. 1999;**83**:514. DOI: 10.1136/bjo.83.5.514

[11] Podgor MJ, Remaley NA, Chew E. Associations between siblings for esotropia and exotropia. Archives of Ophthalmology. 1996;**114**:739. DOI: 10.1001/archopht.1996.01100130731018

[12] Aurell E, Norrsell K. A longitudinal study of children with a family history of strabismus: factors determining the incidence of strabismus. The British Journal of Ophthalmology. 1990;**74**:589. DOI: 10.1136/bjo.74.10.589

[13] Damms T, Damms C, Schulz E, Haase W. Pseudo-esotropia caused by nasal dislocation of the macula in patients with high infantile myopia. Der Ophthalmologe. 1994;**91**:77

[14] Hutchinson AK. Intermittent exotropia. Ophthalmology Clinics of North America. 2001;**14**(3):399-406. DOI: 10.1016/s0896-1549(05)70237-6

[15] McManaway JW III, Frankel CA. Strabismus. In: Primary Pediatric Care.

Hoekelman RA, editor. St. Louis: Mosby; 2001. p. 1253

[16] Coats DK, Paysse EA, Kim DS. Excessive blinking in childhood: a prospective evaluation of 99 children. Ophthalmology. 2001;**108**(9):1556-1561. DOI: 10.1016/s0161-6420(01)00644-3

[17] Kushner BJ, Morton GV. Distance/near differences in intermittent exotropia. Archives of Ophthalmology. 1998;**116**(4):478-486. DOI: 10.1001/archopht.116.4.478

[18] Konjevoda S, Boergen KP, urednici. Dječja oftlamologija i strabologija. Zadar: Sveučilište u Zadru; 2018

[19] Pigassou R. Prisms in strabismus. International Ophthalmology Clinics. 1966;**6**:519

[20] Véronneau-Troutman S. Fresnel prism membrane in the treatment of strabismus. Canadian Journal of Ophthalmology. 1971;**6**:249

[21] Weiss JB, Rouchy JP, Ruellan YM, Teliques JP. Utilisation des prismes compensateurs provisoires pour rompre le circle vicieux "de´viation diplopie.". Belgian Societies of Ophthalmology. 1969;**69**:303

[22] Barrett BT. A critical evaluation of the evidence supporting the practice of behavioural vision therapy. Ophthalmic & Physiological Optics. 2009;**29**(1):4-25. DOI: 10.1111/j.1475-1313.2008.00607.x

[23] Rawstron JA, Burley CD, Elder MJ. A systematic review of the applicability and efficacy of eye exercises. Journal of Pediatric Ophthalmology and Strabismus. 2005;**42**(2):82-88. DOI: 10.3928/01913913-20050301-02

[24] Arnoldi K, Reynolds JD. A review of convergence insufficiency: what are we really accomplishing with exercises? The American Orthoptic Journal. 2007;**57**:123-130. DOI: 10.3368/aoj.57.1.123

[25] Chen AM, Erzurum SA, Chandler DL, et al. Overminus lens therapy for children 3 to 10 years of age with intermittent exotropia: a randomized clinical trial. JAMA Ophthalmology. 2021;**139**(4):464-476. DOI: 10.1001/jamaophthalmol.2021.0082

[26] Pediatric Eye Disease Investigator Group; Mohney BG, Cotter SA, et al. A Randomized trial comparing part-time patching with observation for intermittent exotropia in children 12 to 35 months of age. Ophthalmology. 2015;**122**(8):1718-1725. DOI: 10.1016/j.ophtha.2015.04.025

[27] Pediatric Eye Disease Investigator Group, Cotter SA, Mohney BG, et al. A randomized trial comparing part-time patching with observation for children 3 to 10 years of age with intermittent exotropia. Ophthalmology. 2014;**121**(12):2299-2310. DOI: 10.1016/j.ophtha.2014.07.021

[28] Joyce KE, Beyer F, Thomson RG, Clarke MP. A systematic review of the effectiveness of treatments in altering the natural history of intermittent exotropia. The British Journal of Ophthalmology. 2015;**99**(4):440-450. DOI: 10.1136/bjophthalmol-2013-304627

[29] Duckman RH. Management of binocular anomalies: efficacy of vision therapy, exotropia. American Journal of Optometry and Physiological Optics. 1987;**64**(6):421-429

[30] Convergence Insufficiency Treatment Trial Study Group. Randomized clinical trial of treatments for symptomatic convergence insufficiency in children. Archives of

Ophthalmology. 2008;**126**(10):1336-1349. DOI: 10.1001/archopht.126.10.1336

[31] Wallace DK. Treatment options for symptomatic convergence insufficiency. Archives of Ophthalmology. 2008;**126**(10):1455-1456. DOI: 10.1001/archopht.126.10.1455

[32] Baker JD, Schweers M, Petrunak J. Is earlier surgery a sensory benefit in the treatment of intermittent exotropia? In: Lennerstrand G, editor. Advances in Strabismology. Proceedings of the Eighth Meeting of the International Strabismological Association, Maastricht, Dept. 10-12, 1998. Buren, The Netherlands: Aeolus Press; 1999. p. 289

[33] Ing MR, Nishimura J, Okino L. Outcome study of bilateral lateral rectus recession for intermittent exotropia in children. Transactions of the American Ophthalmological Society. 1997;**95**:433-443 discussion 443-52

[34] Burian HM, editor. Selected problems in the diagnosis and treatment of the neuromuscular anomalies of the eyes. In: II Curso Internacional de Oftalmologia. Barcelona: Publicaciones del Instituto Barranquer; 1958. p. 25

[35] Burian HM, Spivey BE. The surgical management of exodeviations. American Journal of Ophthalmology. 1965;**59**:603

[36] von Noorden GK. Divergence excess and simulated divergence excess: diagnosis and surgical management. Ophthalmologica. 1969;**26**:719

[37] Kushner BJ. Selective surgery for intermittent exotropia based on distance/near differences. Archives of Ophthalmology. 1998;**116**(3):324-328. DOI: 10.1001/archopht.116.3.324

[38] Lange W, de Decker W. Two therapeutic concepts in intermittent divergent squint. Documenta Ophthalmologica. 1993;**84**:187

[39] Yuksel D, Spiritus M, Vandelannoitte S. Chirurgie syme´-trique comme traitement initial de l'exotropie intermittente de base. Bulletin of the Belgian Society of Ophthalmology. 1998;**268**:195-199

[40] Donahue SP. Clinical practice. Pediatric strabismus. The New England Journal of Medicine. 2007;**356**(10):1040-1047. DOI: 10.1056/NEJMcp051888

[41] Buck D, Powell CJ, Sloper JJ, et al. Surgical intervention in childhood intermittent exotropia: current practice and clinical outcomes from an observational cohort study. The British Journal of Ophthalmology. 2012;**96**(10):1291-1295. DOI: 10.1136/bjophthalmol-2012-301981

[42] Hardesty HH, Boynton JR, Keenan JP. Treatment of intermittent exotropia. Archives of Ophthalmology. 1978;**96**(2):268-274. DOI: 10.1001/archopht.1978.03910050136006

[43] Fletcher MC, Silverman SJ, Strabismus I. A summary of 1110 consecutive cases. American Journal of Ophthalmology. 1966;**61**(1):86-94

[44] Laws HW. An evaluation of the use of prisms in the postoperative orthoptic care of divergence strabismus. In: Arruga A, editor. International Strabismus Symposium. University of Giessen, Germany, 1966. Basel: S Karger; 1968. p. 324

[45] Dunlap EA, editor. Overcorrections in horizontal strabismus surgery. In: Symposium on Strabismus. Transactions of the New Orleans Academy of Ophthalmology. St Louis: Mosby–Year Book; 1971. p. 255

[46] Hardesty HH. Treatment of overcorrected intermittent exotropia. American Journal of Ophthalmology. 1968;**66**(1):80-86. DOI: 10.1016/0002-9394(68)91792-3

[47] Dawson ELM, Marshman WE, Lee JP. Role of botulinum toxin A in surgically overcorrected exotropia. American Association for Pediatric Ophthalmology and Strabismus. 1999;**5**:269-271. DOI: 10.1016/s1091-8531(99)70021-2

Chapter 5

Non-Surgical Strabismus Treatment

Alena Kolomytskaya

Abstract

Treatment of strabismus should begin with non-surgical treatments such as visual acuity enhancement through optical correction, amblyopia treatment, prismatic correction, and orthoptic exercises. The goals of the treatment are to align the eyes in cases of accommodative strabismus, improve visual acuity, improve asthenopic problems, and preserve or restore function of binocular vision, when possible. The best way is to eliminate the causes that led to the development of strabismus.

Keywords: strabismus, binocular vision, amblyopia, optical correction, orthoptic exercises

1. Introduction

In the treatment of strabismus, several goals are distinguished: one of the most important is the preservation, development, or restoration of binocular vision especially in children, cosmetic effect, correction of ocular torticollis, increase in eye mobility, elimination of double vision and increase in the field of vision in patients with esotropia. Non-surgical treatments for strabismus include optical correction of refractive errors, treatment of amblyopia, and orthoptic exercises.

2. Correction of refractive error and amblyopia treatment

Strabismus in children leads to inability to the development of binocular vision, which normally provides an assessment of the relative position of objects in space. The basis of binocular vision is normal anatomy, the correct interaction of work between the sensory and motor parts of both eyes together with normal functioning of the visual part of the brain [1].

Motor balance is necessary to work in synergy with sensory fusion and to provide the ability to physically move the eyes in the direction of an object being viewed [2]. Motor imbalance can be caused by anomalies of the extraocular muscles and anomalies of accommodation. These abnormalities make it difficult to hold the eye in a straight position [3].

The sensory part implements the function of binocular vision, the ability of the visual part of the brain to merge two images (from two eyes) into one image [4]. A qualitative characteristic of binocular vision are three stages of binocularity with final result of stereoscopic vision of an object, which allows one to determine the place of an object in space, with depth and volume [5, 6].

IntechOpen

To form normal binocular vision, the eyes must see well, with normal motility, properly positioned, looking in the same direction, and properly focused on the same object, the normal functional ability of the retina, conductive pathways, and higher visual centers is required, on the retina of the same size images in both eyes [5, 7].

Strabismus can occur as an imbalance of sensory and motor parts. Impairments in the sensory region prevent the formation of a clear image on the retina.

Causes of sensory imbalance include refractive errors, differences in the anatomical and optical structure of both eyes (anisometropia), a sharp decrease in visual acuity, or blindness in one eye as a result of trauma or surgical procedures, as well as improper correction of refractive errors [3, 5].

When visual acuity is poor or one eye is blind, deviation can occur due to a lack of stimulus for fusion [8]. The cause of strabismus can be diseases affecting the eye or nervous system (for example, tumors), and injuries in any structures and processes that are involved in the process of visual perception and oculomotor control [3]. A small percentage of strabismus is the result of genetic syndromes, acquired stroke, or disease affecting the extraocular muscles or their innervation [3, 8].

In children, the occurrence of strabismus is accompanied by a complex functional restructuring of the binocular visual system to adapt it to work with an asymmetrical position of the eyes. Children with strabismus use the image of only one eye; the image of the second eye is blocked by the brain, which is invisible to the person himself [7, 9]. Adults usually cannot adapt new situation and struggle with double vision.

Strabismus is divided into concomitant (esotropia, exotropia, vertical) (hypotropia or hypertropia), non-concomitant and paralytic forms.

Treatment should begin immediately as soon as strabismus is detected [10].

The method of complex treatment of strabismus consists of the optical correction of ametropia, amblyopia control, surgeries on the oculomotor muscles, and preoperative and postoperative orthoptic exercises [6, 11–13]. By forcing the brain to use the deviated eye, the visual cortex responsible for that eye receives additional visual stimulation, which allows it to restore or develop a normal level of vision [6].

2.1 Optical correction of refractive error

Treatment of strabismus begins with optical correction of refractive errors: hypermetropia, myopia, and astigmatism to increase visual acuity. For treatment, glasses are prescribed for constant wear and if necessary, occlusion to treat amblyopia [3, 14–17].

Any significant degree of ametropia must be corrected, and in the presence of strabismus, correction of any degree of ametropia is recommended [7, 18]. Before prescription of glasses, children with strabismus or suspected strabismus should undergo cycloplegia to determine the true refraction without the influence of accommodation [13].

Because of long cycloplegic effect that can be amblyopic atropin is not the first choice for diagnostic cycloplegia anymore. The first choice today in pediatric ophthalmology opraxis are cyclopšentolate and tropicamid. For children under one year of age or children with neurological problems, a 1% solution of tropicamide is a method of choice. Tropicamide is instilled 3x times every 15 minutes before the examination. For children older than 1 year, 1% solution of cyclopentolate is usually used. Cyclopentolate is instilled twice with an interval of 10 minutes directly on the day of the examination. Refraction is examined approximately 30–40 minutes after instillation. However, tropicamide does not provide complete cycloplegia, and therefore its use is limited. For children less than 1 year of age, a 0.5% solution of cyclopentolate or a 0.5% solution of tropicamide can be used [7, 18].

When measuring refraction in very young children usually under the age of 3 years, autorefractometers cannot be used and retinoscopy in cycloplegia has to be performed. Rules for refraction prescription depend on the age of the child and type of strabismus. Although for children under 6 years of age, full refractive correction is not necessary in the cases of strabismus usually is recommended [18].

With esotropia, a complete amount of cycloplegic hypermetropia must be fully corrected with glasses even if the amount of hypermetropia is only physiological hypermetropia. Adjusting to full cycloplegic correction in glasses may require some time for relaxation and accommodation. Full correction of hyperopia should be prescribed to eliminate the influence of accommodative convergence. In particular, accommodative esotropia, which is most common in children, is well corrected by constantly wearing properly selected glasses, which leads to correction of eye position, improved vision, and the development of binocularity [19–21]. Although, according to some reports wearing complete cycloplegic hypermetropic correction in children can prevent the development of emmetropia of the eyeball [22], insufficient correction can lead to decompensation of esotropia [21].

For variable exotropia, correction of hyperopia also sometimes has a beneficial effect on exodeviation control and improves binocular status in some patients while complete correction enables the patient to have better accommodation and control of the deviation [6].

Astigmatism of even 1.0 D can reduce visual acuity and cause visual discomfort.

When correcting myopia, it is necessary to strive to ensure clear visualization of distant objects for school children. In younger children, sometimes, myopia does not have to be correct in full amount because their vision is developing at near. In the cases of exotropia, full amount of cycloplegic refraction has to be corrected.

Spectacle correction is necessary after the surgical treatment.

Bifocal glasses are indicated for children with high AC/A coefficient (accommodative ratio of convergence and accommodation) and accommodative esotropia with convergence excess. The upper part of bifocals helps align the eyes at distance and lower part with addition corrects residual excess of esotropia at near. It is obligatory to prescribe a full addition of +3,0 in the beginning and then gradually wean off. The dividing strip in bifocal glasses has to pass in through the middle of the pupil in children. The recommended strategy is to continuously and gradually reduce bifocal correction until the patients restore normal accommodation. In some cases, surgery is needed. The AC/A ratio decreases with age [2].

If patients have amblyopia, treatment begins with amblyopia treatment.

Amblyopia is a decrease in best-corrected visual acuity in one or less often two eyes. It is a developmental disorder of the visual system in some cases accompanied by structural changes in the eye [16]. It develops at an early age, as a result of suppression of the image from the deviated eye, or eye with uncorrected refractive error, or some kind of anatomical disorder (cataract, ptosis, hemangioma), the part of cortex responsible for interpreting the images coming from eye does not receive the stimulation necessary for normal development. As a result of untreated amblyopia, the affected eye develops lower visual acuity due to the abnormal development of the cortical visual pathway or abnormal binocular interactions [23–26].

During occlusion, especially long-term, it is necessary to monitor the visual acuity of the dominant eye, since if it is turned off for a long time, visual acuity may decrease. In such cases, they switch to alternating occlusion.

In some cases when compliance is not good, instead of occlusion, the technique of blurring the image of the eye with better visual acuity can be used. In such cases, atropine penalization and filters are prescribed. These methods are used less frequently but are also useful [14, 16, 26, 27]. Penalization is effective if the vision of the better-seeing eye under conditions of penalization is lower than the visual acuity of the amblyopic eye.

To stimulate the retina of an amblyopic eye, light-color stimulation, the use of reflected laser beams, frequency-contrast stimulation, and electromagnetic stimulation are used. However, the gold standard treatment for amblyopia is correction of the refractive error and occlusion of the better eye [28, 29]. In children, the time of occlusion depends on degree of amblyopia and age of the child (usually, day from 2 to 6 hours). Occlusions are sometimes reasonable in adults [30].

Inverse occlusion therapy is sometimes useful for elimination of inhibition of central fixation to change excentric fixation pattern of squinting eye which can improve control of some forms of strabismus.

Newer binocular treatments for amblyopia are being developed based on neural tasks and games that complement occlusion. Virtual reality is a relatively new intervention that can be used to treat eye and vision problems [21, 31]. Home video therapy can provide patch-equivalent treatment results [32–35].

This therapy involves visual tasks that are designed so that they can only be completed using both eyes. These range from simple games using red-green glasses to exciting 3D games and movies [27, 28, 32, 34, 36].

The exercises are interesting for both children and adults and require active participation on their part. Computer games have a complex effect on various types of visual sensitivity: light, brightness, frequency-contrast, various semantic content, and form, which significantly increase the effectiveness of treatment [7].

Virtual reality depends on software and application design features [31].

Currently, asynchronous stimulation of two eyes is being developed, when visual stimuli are presented to the better-seeing eye with some temporary short-term delay, which leads to a change in eye dominance [24].

Amblyopia treatment should be monitored by an ophthalmologist or orthoptist and the schedule adjusted according to the improvement of the visual acuity. Refraction also changes with age, and examinations are recommended every six months [18]. All children are born hypermetropes because of their small eyes. During the childhood, eyes are developing and growing hypermetropia always decreases, and in adolescence, children with hypermetropia of less than 2.5 D become emmetropes.

Although children tolerate anisometropia much better than adult patients if there is a significant anisometropia and aniseikonia (refractive asymmetry between the eyes) of more than 5 D, it is reasonable to use contact lenses for correction [37–39]. Excimer laser surgery should not be performed until the age of at least 18 years.

If the patient has refractive error, especially in combination with hyperopia and convergent strabismus, as a preoperative preparation, it is mandatory to prescribe glasses for constant wear to correct full cycloplegic refractive error, to identify non-accommodative deviation angle. In the process of presurgical preparation, the accommodative nature of strabismus is revealed. In the cases of accommodative refractive strabismus, after the correction of the full refractive error angle of deviation decreases and the need for surgical correction of strabismus disappears, residual angle after the correction has to be treated surgicaly. Therefore, the accommodative part of squinting angle has to be treated with refractive and not strabismus surgery. If patients do not want to wear glasses in adult age, refractive surgery is always an option for accommodative part.

If children and young people refuse to wear glasses, we recommend that they switch to contact lens correction. But usually, if there is good compliance with the patient and his parents, an explanation of the reasons, and the possible result, patients agree to wear glasses until they reach an age when refractive surgery is possible.

2.2 Orthoptic exercises

Treatment is aimed at restoring (forming) binocular functions. The principle of separating the eyes using mechanical, color and other types of visual field separation and training the patient to combine two images into one image with a gradual transition from artificial to natural conditions is used [7, 40].

The exercises are aimed at improving eye mobility, eliminating abnormal retinal correspondence, and restoring normal relationships between accommodation and convergence [41]. Orthoptic treatment does not affect the angle of the strabismus.

Orthoptic exercises may help a group of patients with good fusion potential by teaching patients how to use their fusion abilities more effectively. To obtain the effect of binocular exercises, visual acuity of the worse-seeing eye is desirable not lower than 0.3–0.4 (20/50) [7].

The exercises help a group of patients with exotropia and convergence insufficiency by objectively improving binocular function after fusion exercises [20, 40, 42]. The effectiveness of home-based pencil push-up therapy has worked well in the treatment of convergence insufficiency.

Wearing complete cycloplegic optical correction in combination with orthoptic exercises can help treat accommodative strabismus [43].

The effectiveness of orthoptic exercises in treating other forms of strabismus is debated. A comprehensive review of the evidence supporting orthoptic exercise/vision therapy conducted in the UK found that there was little evidence-based research to support these practices [43–45].

In post-Soviet countries, synaptophore is used for therapeutic orthoptic exercises, teaching haploscopic vision. The purpose of such exercises is to treat functional scotoma and restore joint functioning of the eyes. However, this vision differs from vision in natural conditions. Under natural conditions, retinal images of the same object merge, and on the synaptophore, images of two objects presented separately for each eye merge. Therefore, it is more expedient to carry out treatment to restore binocular functions without mechanical separation of the visual fields after achieving a symmetrical position of the eyes.

When using games in virtual reality, the conditions are closer to natural, and the games themselves are much more interesting, allowing them to maintain attention and concentration, especially in children. These methods are used with two eyes open, most often by separating the eyes using color filters.

There is also a method of phase haploscopy using liquid crystal glasses. In a certain frequency-phase mode, an electrical pulse passes through the plates of such glasses, changing their transparency: one glass becomes transparent; the other at this moment becomes opaque. Since this change in transparency occurs with high frequency, the patient does not feel it.

In glasses with an autonomous power system, the binocular phase is also turned on, when both eyes look through transparent glass, bringing the patient closer to natural conditions of perception. This treatment method is also used to treat amblyopia, however, due to the high cost of such glasses, the treatment method is not widespread [7].

2.3 Correction with prisms

The use of prisms is an important treatment modality for the management of patients with binocular dysfunction (asthenopia, diplopia). The use of prisms sometimes helps eliminate diplopia in case of small paresis of the eye muscles, reduce or eliminate the compensatory position of the head (torticollis), and help restore binocular vision during the treatment of concomitant strabismus [4]. Prismatic correction is used to eliminate residual small angles after surgical treatment [46], treatment of asthenopia caused by heterophoria [47]. Sometimes good effects can be obtained with prismatic glasses in cases of microesophoria or microtropia [48]. The use of prisms is contraindicated in the absence of symptoms of binocular function and if there is a risk of aggravation of the existing condition in the process of adaptation to fusion.

Prism correction is used to eliminate double vision in two main directions of vision: straight ahead and vertical.

The prism shifts the image towards the base and thus shifts the gaze in the direction of the top of the prism. This effect is used in cases of limited mobility, which is used in the treatment of paretic strabismus [4]. Thus, prisms do not change the position of the eyes; they change the path of rays from the object in question in the eye, affecting sensorimotor relations.

Fresnel prisms are thin flexible plates made of flexible transparent plastic and are attached to ordinary diopter glasses on the back surface of the spectacle glass. Fresnel prisms do not weigh down the glasses. However, there are still some limitations with diminishing visual acuity: the optimally tolerated correction is up to $\leq$20 D. Long-term wearing leads to successful treatment in 30% of cases [49]. Prisms with a small diopter value can be prescribed to the dominant eye.

One prism diopter corresponds to approximately 0.5° (34″) deviation. Prisms are drawn according to the full (360°) TABO scale, and the direction of the base of the prism is always indicated. If there are horizontal and vertical components of deviation, you can separately indicate the strength of the horizontal and vertical prism for each eye, or you can indicate the resulting prism force, which can be calculated on special websites or using tables.

When restoring impaired functions, prismatic correction should gradually decrease with their subsequent abolition. Some authors report that staged prismatic treatment, with a reduction in the power of the prisms used can lead to good results as a treatment in patients with acute esotropia of 25 D or less [50].

Permanent prismatic correction is reserved for elderly patients and in the absence of functional dynamics.

Contraindications for wearing prisms are subjective intolerance to prisms, an increase in the angle of deviation, or increased diplopia under the prism.

3. Conclusions

Non-surgical treatment methods are effective as a treatment for some types of strabismus such as accommodative strabismus, paretic strabismus, and small-angle strabismus. Non-surgical treatment methods are also used as a preparatory stage before surgical treatment.

Treatment of strabismus is a long process. Correctly chosen tactics for the complex treatment of strabismus start with correctly selected glasses that correct refractive errors, treatment of amblyopia in combination with orthoptic exercises, and, if necessary, wearing prismatic glasses can in some cases achieve satisfactory eye alignment and enable development of binocular vision. Good visual acuity together with the presence of binocular vision helps to keep the eyes in a straight position [27, 51].

Author details

Alena Kolomytskaya
Independent Researcher, Minsk, Belarus

*Address all correspondence to: kolomeo@mail.ru

References

[1] Alekseenko SV, Shkorbatova PY. Features of the organization of visual pathways from the retinas and changes in their activity in early disorders of binocular experience. Neva Horizons–2018: Scientific Materials. In: Conference in Ophthalmologists from the International Participation/S.-Peter. State Pediatrician University/St. Peterburg "Polytechnic Service"; 2018. pp. 134-135 [Article in Russian]

[2] Kim WK, Kang SY, Rhiu S, Chung SA, Lee JB. The analysis of AC/a ratio in nonrefractive accommodative esotropia treated with bifocal glasses. Korean Journal of Ophthalmology. 2012;**26**(1):39-44. DOI: 10.3341/kjo.2012.26.1.39 Epub 2012 Jan 14

[3] Kanukollu VM, Sood G. Strabismus. In: StatPearls [Internet]. Treasure Island (FL): StatPearls Publishing; 2023 2022 Aug 8. Bookshelf ID: NBK560782 Free Books & Documents

[4] Eppenberger LS, Taranto R, Bücheler A, Heckmann J, Sturm V. Prism-induced gaze shift and strabismus treatment for ocular motility disorders and anomalous head posture. Klinische Monatsblätter für Augenheilkunde. 2021;**238**(4):474-477. DOI: 10.1055/a-1407-9437 Epub 2021 Apr 30.[Article in German]

[5] Horwood AM. Why do babies develop strabismus. In: Trasactions of the 39th European Strabismological Association (ESA) Metting, Porto, 13-15 Sept. 2017. Porto: Eur. Strabismol. Assoc.; 2017. pp. 33-40

[6] Kassem IS, Rubin SE, Kodsi SR. Exotropia in children with high hyperopia. Journal of AAPOS. 2012;**16**(5):437-440. DOI: 10.1016/j.jaapos.2012.06.003

[7] Avetisov SE. [et others] Ophthalmology: National Leadership/Society of Ophthalmologists of Russia, Interregional. Association of Ophthalmologists. Moscow: GEOTAR-Media; 2008. 940 p

[8] Sunyer-Grau B, Quevedo L, Rodríguez-Vallejo M, Argilés M. Comitant strabismus etiology: Extraocular muscle integrity and central nervous system involvement-a narrative review. Graefe's Archive for Clinical and Experimental Ophthalmology. 2023;**261**(7):1781-1792. DOI: 10.1007/s00417-022-05935-9 Epub 2023 Jan 21

[9] Economides JR, Adams DL, Horton JC. Perception via the deviated eye in strabismus. The Journal of Neuroscience. 2012;**32**(30):10286-10295. DOI: 10.1523/JNEUROSCI.1435-12.2012

[10] Kashchenko TP, Aklaeva NA. The sequence and tactics of complex treatment of concomitant strabismus. In: Fedorov Readings - 2007: Anniversary. Scientific-Practical. In: Conference on SAT Abstract, Moscow, June 14-15, 2007. Assoc. Ophthalmologists of Russia, MNTK "Eye Microsurgery" named after. S.N.Fedorova, editor. By Takhchidi, Moscow. LLC House of printing "Capital Business"; 2007. pp. 368-369 [Article in Russian]

[11] Arnoldi K, Reynolds JD. A review of convergence insufficiency: What are we really accomplishing with exercises? American Orthoptic Journal. 2007;**57**:123-130

[12] Kikolashvili MS, Shengeliia DG, Tsomaia LV. Treatment of non accomodated concomitant strabismus. Georgian Medical News. 2011;**191**:22-26

[13] Kothari M, Manurung F, Paralkar S. Use of atropine to predict the accommodative component in esotropia with hypermetropia. Indian Journal of Ophthalmology. 2011;**59**(6):487-490. DOI: 10.4103/0301-4738.86319

[14] Ahmed N, Fashner J. Eye conditions in infants and children: Amblyopia and strabismus. FP Essentials. 2019;**484**:18-22

[15] Writing Committee for the Pediatric Eye Disease Investigator Group, Cotter SA, Foster NC, Holmes JM, Melia BM, Wallace DK, et al. Optical treatment of strabismic and combined strabismic-anisometropic amblyopia. Ophthalmology. 2012;**119**(1):150-158. DOI: 10.1016/j.ophtha.2011.06.043 Epub 2011 Sep 29

[16] Nentwich MM. Amblyopia-basic principles and current diagnostic and therapeutic standards. Der Ophthalmologe. 2019;**116**(4):391-404. DOI: 10.1007/s00347-019-0876-4

[17] Popova NA, Meluzova RD. Features of refraction and results of treatment of patients with congenital fibrosis syndrome of extraocular muscles. In: Fedorov Readings - 2008: Sat. Scientific Art. VII all-Russian. Scientific-Practical. In: Conference with International Participation. Moscow, MNTK "Eye Microsurgery" named after. acad. S.N.Fedorova; ed. by Takhchidi, Moscow. LLC House of printing "Capital Business"; 2008. pp. 90-91 [Article in Russian]

[18] Kanski JJ. Clinical Ophthalmology. Moscow/Moscow publishing house "Logosphere"; 2006. 744 p [in Russian]

[19] Kononova NE, Somov EE. Features of the functional state of the organ of vision in children with various types of concomitant strabismus neva horizons–2018: Scientific materials. In: Conference in Ophthalmologists from the International Participation/S.-Peter. State Pediatrician University/St. Peterburg "Polytechnic Service"; 2018. pp. 149-151 [Article in Russian]

[20] Lembo A, Serafino M, Strologo M, Saunders RA, Trivedi RH, Villani E, et al. Accommodative esotropia: The state of the art. International Ophthalmology. 2019;**39**(2):497-505. DOI: 10.1007/s10792-018-0821-6 Epub 2018 Jan 13

[21] Zhao C, Wei Y. Optical correction principles of accommodative esotropia. Zhonghua Yan Ke Za Zhi. 2021;**57**(5):331-335. DOI: 10.3760/cma.j.cn112142-20210202-00071

[22] Sefi-Yurdakul N, Kaykısız H, Koç F. The effects of partial and full correction of refractive errors on sensorial and motor outcomes in children with refractive accommodative esotropia. International Ophthalmology. 2019;**39**(4):883-890. DOI: 10.1007/s10792-018-0889-z Epub 2018 Mar 17

[23] Helveston EM. Understanding, detecting, and managing strabismus. Community Eye Health. 2010;**23**(72):12-14

[24] Huang X, Xia H, Zhang Q, Blakemore C, Nan Y, Wang W, et al. New treatment for amblyopia based on rules of synaptic plasticity: A randomized clinical trial. Science China Life Sciences. 2022;**65**(3):451-465. DOI: 10.1007/s11427-021-2030-6 Epub 2022 Jan 6

[25] Fan Y, Li L, Chu P, Wu Q, Wang Y, Cao W, et al. Clinical analysis of eye movement-based data in the medical diagnosis of amblyopia. Methods. 2023;**213**:26-32. DOI: 10.1016/j.ymeth.2023.03.003 Epub 2023 Mar 15

[26] Sen S, Singh P, Saxena R. Management of amblyopia in pediatric patients: Current insights. Eye (London, England). 2022;**36**(1):44-56.

DOI: 10.1038/s41433-021-01669-w Epub 2021 Jul 7

[27] Chaturvedi I, Jamil R, Sharma P. Binocular vision therapy for the treatment of amblyopia-a review. Indian Journal of Ophthalmology. 2023;**71**(5):1797-1803. DOI: 10.4103/IJO.IJO_3098_22

[28] Kaur S, Sharda S, Aggarwal H, Dadeya S. Comprehensive review of amblyopia: Types and management. Indian Journal of Ophthalmology. 2023;**71**(7):2677-2686. DOI: 10.4103/IJO.IJO_338_23

[29] Meier K, Tarczy-Hornoch K. Recent treatment advances in amblyopia. Annual Review of Vision Science. 2022;**8**:323-343. DOI: 10.1146/annurev-vision-100720-022550 Epub 2022 Apr 4. Review

[30] Ridder WH, Patel R, Li Y-X, Staubli U. Standard amblyopia therapy in adults with longstanding amblyopia improves visual acuity and contrast sensitivity. Clinical Ophthalmology. 2023;**17**:1847-1858. DOI: 10.2147/OPTH.S410800 eCollection 2023

[31] Chan HS, Tang YM, Do CW, Wong HHY, LYL C, S T. Design and assessment of amblyopia, strabismus, and myopia treatment and vision training using virtual reality. Digit Health. 2023;**9**:20552076231176638. DOI: 10.1177/20552076231176638. eCollection 2023 Jan-Dec

[32] Lee HL, Kim SL. Effectiveness of binocularity-stimulating treatment in children with residual amblyopia following occlusion. BMC Ophthalmology. 2018;**18**(1):253. DOI: 10.1186/s12886-018-0922-z

[33] Poltavski D, Adams RJ, Biberdorf D, Patrie JT. Effectiveness of a novel video game platform in the treatment of Pediatric amblyopia. Journal of Pediatric Ophthalmology and Strabismus. 25 Apr 2023:1-10. DOI: 10.3928/01913913-20230324-01. PMID: 37092663

[34] Tailor V, Bossi M, Bunce C, Greenwood JA, Dahlmann-Noor A. Binocular versus standard occlusion or blurring treatment for unilateral amblyopia in children aged three to eight years. Cochrane Database of Systematic Reviews. 2015;**2015**(8):CD011347. DOI: 10.1002/14651858.CD011347.pub2

[35] Zhu Q, Zhao Q, Liang R, He X, Gao M. Effectiveness of binocular therapy as a complementary treatment of part-time patching in older amblyopic children: A randomized clinical trial. International Ophthalmology. 2023;**43**(7):2433-2445. DOI: 10.1007/s10792-023-02642-0 Epub 2023 Mar 6

[36] Mohan A, Kaur N, Sen P, Jain E, Gajraj M. Efficacy of smartphone-based exercises in conjunction with modified glasses prescription in the treatment of convergence insufficiency and fusion weakness. Journal of Binocular Vision and Ocular Motility. 2019;**69**(1):30-33. DOI: 10.1080/2576117X.2019.1578594 Epub 2019 Mar 1

[37] Gabai A, Zeppieri M. Anisometropia. In: StatPearls [Internet]. Treasure Island. FL: StatPearls Publishing; 2023 2023 May 11

[38] Eustis HS. Shah. Accomodative esotropia treatment plan utilizing simultaneous strabismus surgery and photorefractive keratectomy. American Journal of Ophthalmology. 2018;**187**:125-129. DOI: 10.1016/j.ajo.2018.01.005 Epub 2018 Jan 12

[39] South J, Gao T, Collins A, Turuwhenua J, Robertson K, Black J. Aniseikoniaand anisometropia:Implications for suppression and amblyopia. Clinical & Experimental Optometry.

2019;**102**(6):556-565. DOI: 10.1111/cxo.12881 Epub 2019 Feb 21

[40] Pejic Z, Wong W, Husain R, Ling Y, Farzavandi S. Fusion exercises for treatment of intermittent exotropia and phoria. The American Orthoptic Journal. 2006;**56**:138-146. DOI: 10.3368/aoj.56.1.138

[41] De Ruiter BJ, Kotha VS, Peiffer AJ, Lesko RP, Tannen B, Tannen N, et al. Orthoptic vision therapy: Establishing a protocol for management of diplopia following orbital fracture repair. The Journal of Craniofacial Surgery. 2021;**32**(3):1025-1028. DOI: 10.1097/SCS.0000000000007099

[42] Boon MY, Asper LJ, Chik P, Alagiah P, Ryan M. Treatment and compliance with virtual reality and anaglyph-based training programs for convergence insufficiency. Clinical & Experimental Optometry. 2020;**103**(6):870-876. DOI: 10.1111/cxo.13057 Epub 2020 Mar 22

[43] Aziz S, Cleary M, Stewart HK, Weir CR. Are orthoptic exercises an effective treatment for convergence and fusion deficiencies? Strabismus. 2006;**14**(4):183-189. DOI: 10.3368/aoj.57.1.123

[44] Aznauryan IE, Balasanyan VO, Nikitina AA. Modern system of surgical treatment for various types of horizontal concomitant strabismus in children and adolescents. In: VIII all-Russian Scientific and Practical Conference with International Participation "Fedorov Readings - 2009": Sat. Abstract, Moscow, July 1-3, 2009. Assoc. Ophthalmologists of Russia [and other]; under general ed. Takhchidi, Moscow/ LLC "House of printing "Capital Business"; 2009. pp. 176-177 [Article in Russian]

[45] Ridder WH, Rouse MW. Predicting potential acuities in amblyopes: Predicting post-therapy acuity in amblyopes. Documenta Ophthalmologica. 2007;**114**(3):135-145. DOI: 10.1007/s10633-007-9048-y Epub 2007 Feb 20

[46] Zou YC, Liu L. The management of childhood esotropia with hyperopia. Current Medical Research and Opinion. 2011;**27**(4):731-735. DOI: 10.1185/03007995.2011.552973 Epub 2011 Jan 25

[47] Gray LS. The prescribing of prisms in clinical practice. Graefe's Archive for Clinical and Experimental Ophthalmology. 2008;**246**(5):627-629. DOI: 10.1007/s00417-008-0799-2 Epub 2008 Apr 1

[48] Lee HJ, Kim SJ. Management of patients with small-angle esotropia and subnormal stereopsis using Fresnel prism. Graefe's Archive for Clinical and Experimental Ophthalmology. 2022;**260**(1):345-352. DOI: 10.1007/s00417-021-05338-2 Epub 2021 Aug 18

[49] Choe HR, Yang HK, Hwang JM. Long-term outcomes of prismatic correction in partially accommodative esotropia. PLoS One. 2019;**14**(12):e0225654. DOI: 10.1371/journal.pone.0225654 eCollection 2019

[50] Wu Y, Feng X, Li J, Chang M, Wang J, Yan H. Prismatic treatment of acute acquired concomitant esotropia of 25 prism diopters or less. BMC Ophthalmology. 2022;**22**(1):276. DOI: 10.1186/s12886-022-02501-z

[51] Sharma P, Gaur N, Phuljhele S, Saxena R. What's new for us in strabismus? Indian Journal of Ophthalmology. 2017;**65**(3):184-190

Chapter 6

Treatment of Paralytic Eye Motility Disorders

Ivana Mravicic, Alma Biscevic, Melisa Ahmedbegović Pjano, Ivona Petrovska, Anja Shumejko and Nina Ziga

Abstract

Paralytic strabismus is caused by paresis or paralysis of one or more extraocular muscles that are innervated by cranial nerve lll, IV and Vl. They are characterized by squinting angle that depends on the direction of the gaze and the fixating eye. Typically, the angle is greater in the field of affected muscle, and when the patient is fixing with the affected eye. While younger children in some cases can suppress double vision, older children and adults with acquired paralytic strabismus usually have diplopia, which they try to avoid by compensatory head posture. Some types of paralytic strabismus can be congenital but it is important to diagnose acquired paralytic strabismus that can be caused by some neurological or systemic disorders and requires further investigation. Treatment of the paralytic strabismus is challenging, and despite the multiple surgeries, results can be disappointing.

Keywords: paralytic strabismus, third nerve palsy, sixth nerve palsy, fourth nerve palsy, eye muscle surgeries

1. Introduction

Paralytic strabismus is caused by paresis or paralysis of one or more extraocular muscles. They are characterised by incomitant strabismus with the variable squinting angle that depends on the direction of the gaze and the fixating eye. Typically, the angle is greater in the field of affected muscle, and when the patient is fixing with the affected eye. While younger children can suppress double vision, older children and adults with acquired paralytic strabismus usually have diplopia, which they try to avoid by compensatory head posture (CHP). It is important to distinguish acquired paralytic strabismus from the comitant form. Acquired paralytic form may be caused by some neurological or systemic abnormalities, requires further neurological investigation and can be life threatening. Treatment of paralytic strabismus is challenging, and despite multiple surgeries, results can be disappointing.

2. Third nerve palsy

Oculomotor palsy can be congenital or acquired, complete or partial, pupil-sparing or pupil-involving and isolated or accompanied by neurological conditions [1].

Third nerve palsy in children is usually congenital but can be acquired later as a result of trauma, inflammation or rarely from neoplastic lesions. Congenital palsies are usually secondary to maldevelopment, intrauterine insult or birth trauma. When bilateral, congenital lll nerve palsies are usually a part of congenital cranial dysinnervation disorders (CCDD) in which genetic mutations lead to abnormal development of cranial nerves III, IV and VI, which results in secondary changes of extraocular muscles and development of a complex, incomitant strabismus. Unilateral cases may be a part of neurofibromatosis type II, posterior fossa malformations, septo-optic dysplasia or some other neurological disorders [2]. Among acquired forms, trauma is the most common cause in child's age, trauma and infections together with aneurysms, diabetes or microvascular infarction are more often cause of third nerve palsy in adults. Children can have transient ophthalmoplegia following infection or migraine [3]. The clinical picture should be always correlated with the age and systemic diseases of the patient.

The nuclear complex of oculomotorius nerve lies in the midbrain and each muscle has its own subnucleus [4].

2.1 Subnuclei of III nerve

Levator subnucleus: unpaired nucleus for both levator muscles (lesion causes bilateral ptosis).

Superior rectus nucleus: paired nucleus that are innervating contralateral superior rectus muscle (lesion causes contralateral elevation deficit).

Medial, inferior rectus and inferior oblique muscle subnuclei: paired subnuclei each supply ipsilateral respected muscle.

Visceral nuclei: parasympathetic innervation to sphincter pupillae and ciliary muscle.

Clinical picture can be different depending on which part of the III nerve is involved. In cases of total palsy, position of the affected eye is typically 'down and out', determined by the function of two intact muscles, the lateral rectus and superior oblique muscle. Affected eye will be in abduction, with slight depression and intorsion with ptosis of affected lid and dilated pupil unreactive to light and accommodation (**Figure 1**). Movement deficit will include adduction, elevation and depression with motility possible only in abduction and to small degree in depression with incyclotorsion (action of the superior oblique, which is minor when eye is abducted). Due to relaxation in tonus of four extraocular muscles, a small amount of proptosis can be present. Adult patients or older children will experience diplopia, which can be horizontal, vertical or oblique, depending on the muscle involved. Younger children due to cortical suppression of the image of the deviated eye may not develop double vision. In cases of longstanding palsy, or palsy that is progressing gradually over time, development of aberrant nerve regeneration can take place, which leads sometimes to perplexing clinical picture. Most often misdirection is presented as anomalous lid excursion during the movement of the eye (retraction of the lid during the movement of the eye), or abnormal horizontal or vertical movement during the attempt to move the eye in the field of action of the affected muscle. **Table 1** shows clinical characteristics of complete III nerve palsy.

In cases of partial involvement, any combination of the affected muscles and/or lid and pupil can be involved. Superior division (superior rectus muscle and levator palpebre) or inferior division (rectus superior and medialis, and inferior oblique muscle) can be affected independently. Each of individual muscles can be involved alone or in combination with each other.

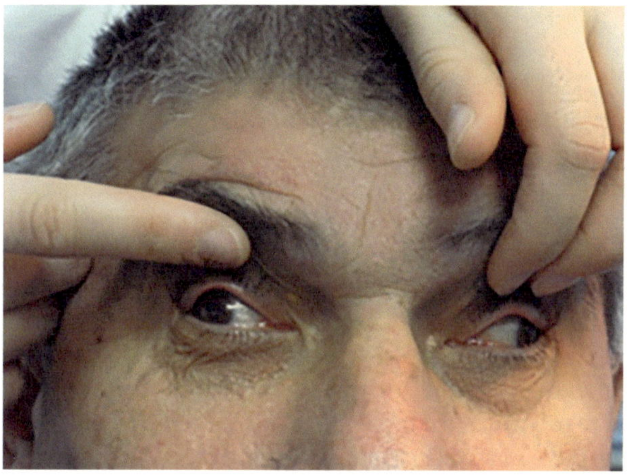

Figure 1.
Clinical picture of bilateral III nerve palsy.

Clinical characterisitcs of the complete III nerve palsy
Eye "out and down", large exotropia with a small hypotropia, intorsion
Ptosis
Fixed and dilated pupil
Reduced: adduction, elevation and depression
Motility: abduction, small amount of depression and incyclotorsion
Compensatory head posture: face turned to the opposite side and chin up

Table 1.
Clinical characteristics of complete III nerve palsy.

After diagnosing the palsy on the basis of clinical picture and history, it is obligatory to continue the investigation of the aetiology. Neurological examination together with imaging (CT and/or MRI) are usually required. In some congenital cases, where diagnosis of palsy is clearly not connected with some progressive neurologic or systemic disease, imaging is not obligatory. Acquired III nerve palsy in children is usually sign of some underlying neurological disease. Associated neurological or systemic signs and symptoms will help examiner to clear etiology of the palsy. The need for repeated imaging is controversial; some suggest that in cases of unclear aetiology, imaging should be repeated after one or two years to exclude some neoplastic or vascular abnormality that was too subtle to be found during the first imaging.

2.2 Differential diagnosis

The diagnosis in the III nerve palsy is usually clear in the cases of complete muscle paresis but can be perplexing in partial palsies when different muscles are involved. Myasthenia gravis or multiple sclerosis can mimic clinical picture of III nerve palsy with lid involvement. Double elevator palsy or orbital floor fracture can have similar clinical picture as superior division palsy.

2.3 Treatment

At child's age, risk of developing amblyopia is high and has to be treated with conservative treatment aggressively and immediately from the beginning, with refractive correction and patching. In congenital cases with no chances for recovery, surgery has to be planned at an early age. In cases of acquired palsy, chances of spontaneous recovery are sometimes good, so surgery should be postponed for at least 6 months. Conservative treatment is based on alleviating double vision with prism correction when possible, or occlusion of the affected eye. Surgery is the method of choice in the cases of acquired, non-progressive palsy that does not improve or resolve during the period of 6–12 months. Surgical approach depends on the muscle involved and extent of the paresis (complete or partial). In cases of complete palsy, often more than one surgery is required with the result that is only partially satisfying in appearance and functionality. In some cases, in early stages, botulinum toxin can be helpful. It is obligatory to talk to the patient before the surgery and explain that operation will not enable normal movement of the eye, but only restore usable field of binocular single vision and achieve acceptable appearance. The type of surgery can vary depending on the muscles involved and amount of action that is present in the affected muscle. Varying from combined recess-resect procedures in supramaximal numbers up to 15 mm. Although in the beginning, results of the surgery are satisfactory the effect of the surgery diminishes over time. Vertical deviation can be improved during the combined horizontal procedure with vertical transposition of horizontal muscles or by performing recession and resection of vertical muscles. Transposition surgeries on SO can be performed in more complicated cases with complete third nerve palsies [5]. Aberrant regeneration improves strabismic deviation but may be complicated to solve during surgical interventions.

Ptosis surgery has to be considered after the strabismus surgeries are completed. The type of intervention depends on levator muscle function (levator resection or frontalis sling surgery) with care taken about the corneal exposure.

3. Sixth nerve palsy

Palsies of the sixth nerve are less common in children but are most often palsies of cranial nerves in adult patients [6]. Typical clinical picture is characterised as an esotropia in primary position (**Figure 2**) with increasing deviation in the field of paretic lateral rectus. The nucleus of nervus abducens is situated in caudal part of pons and innervates lateral rectus muscle on the same side. Fibres of cranial nerve VII loop around the sixth nerve nucleus, therefore, lesions of these two nerves can often occur together.

Children with sixth nerve palsy can develop and preserve binocular vision by adopting compensatory head postures by turning the head in the direction of the affected muscle. Deviation is bigger at distance than near. Congenital sixth nerve palsy in children is rare; however, transient lateral rectus palsy can be present in newborns with spontaneous resolution within 6 weeks. Apart from neurological causes (brain stem pathology, hydrocephalus) or trauma, common cause of 'benign' acquired palsy in early childhood can be isolated sixth nerve palsy related to infectious or immunological process. This kind of postviral inflammatory neuropathy typically has an acute onset 1–3 weeks after viral infection or immunisation [8].

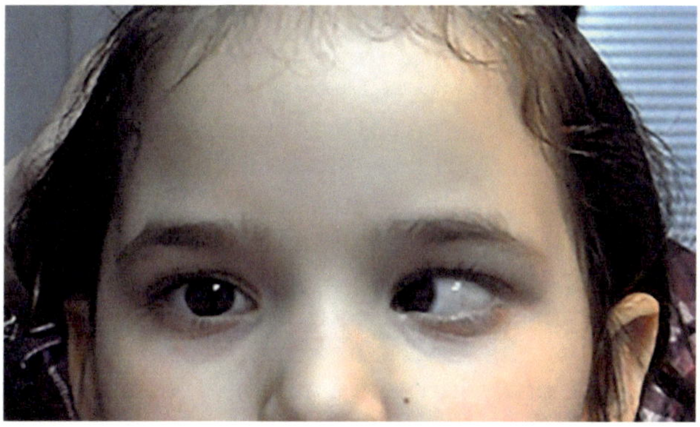

Figure 2.
Clinical picture of VI nerve palsy before and after surgery, (medial rectus recession + Hummelsheim procedure).

These children have to be closely monitored during the improvement, which usually takes 3–6 months. Although recurrences can happen in this kind of palsy, in cases of multiple recurrences or incomplete recovery, additional neurological work up and imaging are recommended to exclude other causes (occult tumour) [9]. In some cases of elevated intracranial pressure, meningitis or excessive trauma sixth nerve palsy can be bilateral. In adult patients, microvascular diseases (diabetes, hypertension or atherosclerosis) together with closed-head trauma are among leading causes. Clinical characteristics of sixth nerve palsy are shown in **Table 2**.

3.1 Differential diagnosis

In newborns, early esotropia syndrome can be misdiagnosed as a congenital sixth nerve palsy. The difference between these two disorders can be made by demonstrating full abduction of the affected eye by doll's head manoeuvre. Duane retraction sy or Mobius sy have impaired abduction but these disorders are presented with restriction rather than limitation, which is manifested by retraction of the globe, narrowing of the lid aperture and an upshot and downshoot in adduction [7].

3.2 Treatment

Conservative treatment includes prevention of amblyopia in child's age. Care should be taken, especially in children who do not turn their heads, because that can indicate suppression of the deviated eye and lead to amblyopia. Refractive error

Clinical characterisitcs of VI nerve palsy
Reduction of abduction on affected eye
Deviation greater at distance than at near
Deviation greater when affected eye is fixing
In unilateral or cases with asymmetry: head turn towards affected side
Esotropia that increases when looking to the affected side

Table 2.
Clinical characteristics of VI nerve palsy.

has to be corrected together with patching of unaffected eye. Majority of cases of acquired abducens palsy will recover during the period of six months. In cases when spontaneous recovery does not occur, surgery is indicated. Surgery depends on amount of action that is present in the affected muscle [10]. In cases of partial palsy when some of the functions are still possible, combined, graded surgery in augmented numbers (recess/resect with calculations based on preserved function) on both horizontal rectus muscles is usually performed. In the cases of complete palsy with no remained function, muscle transposition surgeries are usually method of choice. The full tendon transposition of vertical muscles towards lateral rectus is not a method of choice avoiding the risk of anterior segment ischemia. Therefore, other, more vessel-sparing procedures are commonly used (Hummelsheim, Jensen and different kinds of modifications). In *Hummelsheim* procedure, superior and inferior muscles are split in two halves from the tendon to the 14 mm from the insertion. Temporal parts of both muscles are then sutured adjacent to the insertion of the lateral rectus (**Figure 3**). In *Jensen* procedure (muscle union procedure), muscle bellies of both vertical and lateral muscles are split in half without disinsertion at the insertion. Bellies of vertical muscles are then sutured to the upper and lower half of the lateral muscle approximately 12 mm behind the insertion (**Figure 4**). In *Nishida* procedure, temporal half of vertical muscles are split without disinsertion and fixed to the sclera at the borders of lateral muscle 8 mm posterior to the insertion (**Figure 5**).

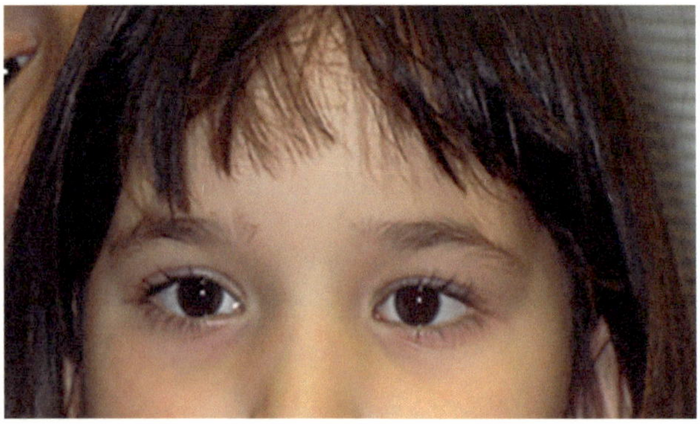

Figure 3.
Hummelsheim procedure.

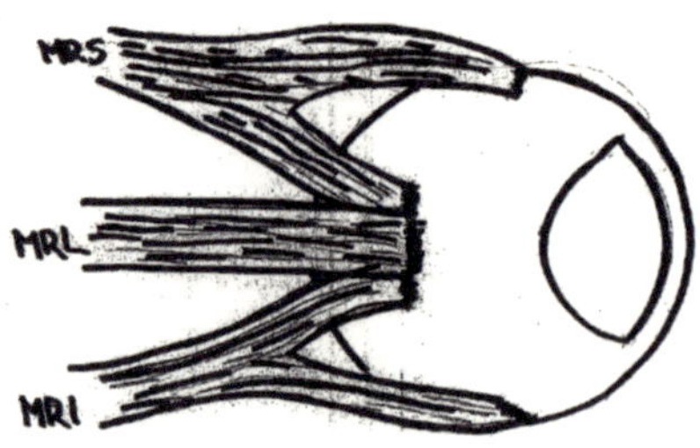

Figure 4.
Jensen procedure.

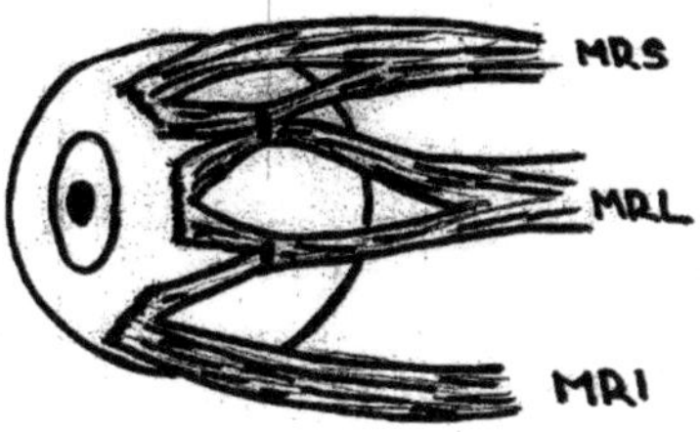

Figure 5.
Nishida procedure.

4. Fourth nerve palsy

Fourth cranial nerve innervates superior oblique muscle. Palsy can be congenital or acquired. Although the term unilateral congenital fourth nerve palsy is widely used in the cases of elevation in adduction in children, some clinical characteristics strongly suggest that not all of the cases with elevation in adduction are fourth nerve palsy. Differences should be noticed between the cases of true palsy where typical signs of paresis, such as increasing deviation in the field of affected muscle, are present, and cases of inferior oblique overaction (IOOA) where the deviation is same in different gaze directions (no incomitance). In non-paretic cases, the deviation should be classified as IOOA or strabismus sursoaductorius (**Figure 6**). In the cases of IOOA despite marked vertical deviation, patients do not complain of diplopia except in the cases of decompensation. However, in some congenital cases, signs of incomitance are present or/and signs of muscle absence or not fully developed superior oblique muscle are found on imaging. Therefore, these cases are truly congenital cases of superior oblique muscle palsy. Clinical differences between IOOA and congenital fourth nerve palsy are presented in **Table 3**. The distinction between congenital and acquired palsy

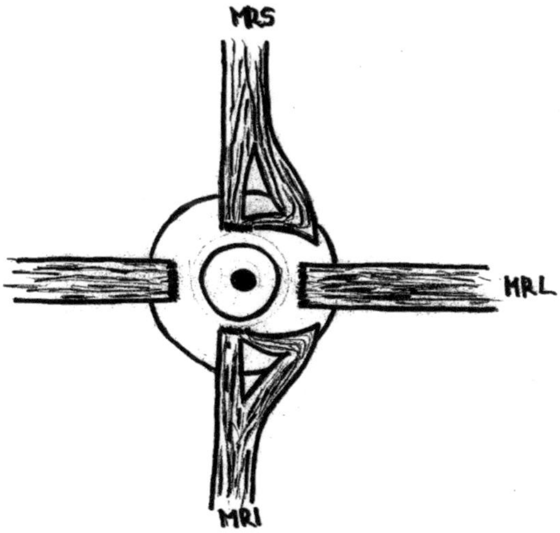

Figure 6.
Differences in clinical picture between fourth nerve palsy and IOOA (CHP).

Clinical features	IOOA (or strabismus sursoaductorius)	Trochlear palsy
History (old photo)	Head tilt or turn	Negative
Onset	Intermittent	Sudden
Vertical deviaton	Comitant in adduction	Maximum in down gaze
Cyclotropic deviation	Small, comittant	Maximum in down gaze
Elevation in adduction	Marked	Negative
Vertical fusional amplitude	Enlarged (up to 15 PD)	Normal (2-3 PD)
Beilschowsky head tilt test	Same in up, pp and down gaze	Maximum in down gaze
Facial asymmetry	Fuller face of the affected side	Negative

Table 3.
Differences in clinical picture between strabismus sursoaductorius (IOOA) and unilateral acquired fourth nerve palsy.

is important because recently diagnosed palsy can be result of intracranial lesion and requires neurologic investigation [11].

Acquired cases are more common in adults. Most common causes are closed-head trauma, vascular lesions and intracranial tumours. In cases of traumatic origin, paralysis is often bilateral but asymmetrical. The main clinical sign is excyclotropia, which increases in downgaze. Motility testing reveals under action of affected superior oblique muscle and in some cases, overaction of inferior oblique muscle. Vertical deviation has to be measured in pp, up and down gaze, with amount of deviation larger when eyes are in infraversion. In bilateral cases, V pattern is present. The amount of cyclotorsion is large and increases in downgaze. It can be measured with Madox rod test. However, for measurement of cyclotorsion, as well as vertical and horizontal deviation in the field of 25°–30° of primary positions, the Harms Tangent screen has to be used whenever possible. Torsion can be confirmed by fundus photography. Vertical and torsional double vision are usually present and increasing in the field of action of the affected muscle. In unilateral cases, compensatory head posture is head tilt on other shoulder, sometimes with chin down (**Figure 7**). Some asymmetric bilateral cases tend to look like unilateral palsy, so care should be taken to confirm if both sides are affected. Bilateral palsies are often in the cases of blunt trauma. When both muscles are affected, patient has marked cyclotropia that is greater in downgaze, with tilted double vision in infraduction and chin up as a compensatory position.

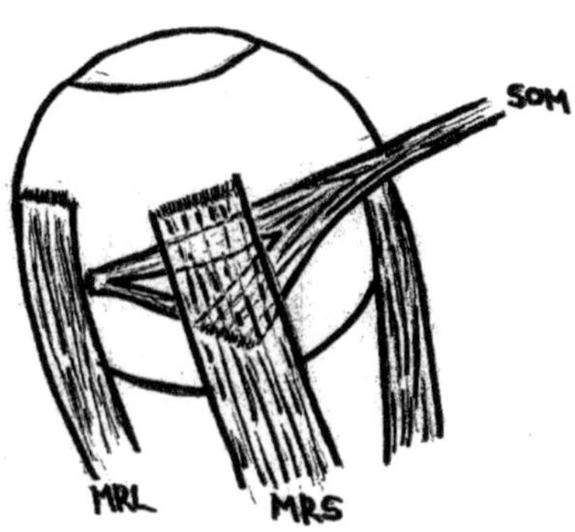

Figure 7.
Harada–Ito procedure.

4.1 Differential diagnosis

Strabismus sursoaductiorius (IOOA) is most common differential diagnosis, especially in congenital cases. In some cases, contralateral superior rectus muscle weakness or DVD on affected eye can have similar clinical symptoms as fourth nerve palsy.

4.2 Treatment

Treatment of underlying disease when possible is first step. In the cases of palsy when underlying disease is not found or not possible to treat, waiting for possible recovery at least six months is recommended. To alleviate torsional double vision, patching of affected eye is often required. Most often complaint that needs correction in patients with acquired fourth nerve palsy is torsion, which can exceed 15° in bilateral cases. Since these deviations cannot be compensated with prism correction, and down gaze is needed functionally in everyday's activities (reading, eating), surgery is the best method of choice. Surgical treatment depends on the clinical picture. Since excyclotorsion in down gaze is most prominent obstacle to fusion, it has to be addressed first. In the Harada–Ito procedure, anterior part of superior oblique muscle is pulled laterally and anteriorly to the upper border of the lateral rectus (in the direction of muscle action), which is the best choice to correct cyclotorsion. Some modifications of this method (Fells or Boergen modification) are recommended in order to increase the effect on cyclodeviation. Since the anterior part is not detached from the muscle, this kind of surgery will have effect on vertical and horizontal deviation in adduction as well (**Figure 7**) [12].

In the cases where this kind of surgery is not sufficient, or vertical deviation is more than 5°, additional tuck of posterior part of the superior oblique tendon or combined surgery on oblique muscles can be performed. While this kind of surgery affects predominantly excyclotorsion, which is usually the major problem, especially in bilateral cases, sometimes in monocular cases, when vertical deviation is predominant, transposition of LR and MR downwards can be method of choice.

5. Conclusion

Paralytic eye motility disorders are complex groups of eye motility problems that can be caused by many reasons. Some of the cases are herited, with the possibility to identify the locus that is responsible for the motility impairment, but unfortunately for the time being there is no genetic treatment available. In many cases, motility problems are caused by neurological diseases. Since some neurological diseases can be life-threatening, we have to be well-coordinated with neurologists. Neurological treatment or sometimes neurosurgical treatment can, in some cases, solve problem with eye motility. However, even with help of other specialists and/or conservative ophthalmological treatment, we often have to treat these patients surgically. Surgical approach is often more complex and demanding than treatment in other kinds of strabismus and results are less satisfactory. Surgery has to be the last option, usually after at least six months after the motility problem starts to be sure that possible spontaneous recovery will not take place. In cases of paretic muscles, it is reasonable whenever possible to prefer recessions more than resections to improve mobility. In the cases of total paralysis and good function of other muscles, muscle transposition can also be method of choice. Last but not the least, it is important to talk with patients and try to explain that with surgical treatment, we cannot restore muscle function, but can improve position of the eye, and by that improve double vision and compensatory head position.

Author details

Ivana Mravicic[1]*, Alma Biscevic[2], Melisa Ahmedbegović Pjano[3], Ivona Petrovska[2], Anja Shumejko[2] and Nina Ziga[2]

1 Eye Clinic Svjetlost, Zagreb, Croatia

2 Ophthalmology Eye Clinic 'Svjetlost', University of Rijeka Medical School, Zagreb, Croatia

3 Eye Clinic Svjetlost, Sarajevo, Bosnia and Herzegovina

*Address all correspondence to: ivana.mravicic@svjetlost.hr

References

[1] Chugh JP, Prachi J, Chouhan RS, Rathi A. Third nerve palsy: An overview. Indian Journal of Clinical Practice. 2012;**22**(12):17-20

[2] Zak R, Slamovits T, Burde R. Oculomotor brainstem anatomy: Nuclei to fascicles. Journal of Neuro-Oncology. 1994;**18**(3):241-248

[3] Carlow TJ. Oculomotor ophthalmoplegic migraine: Is it really migraine. Journal of Neuro-Ophthalmology. 2002;**22**(3):215-221

[4] Umapathi T, Koon SW, Mukkam RP, Chin LS, Beng TC, Helen T, et al. Insights into three dimensional structure of the oculomotor nuclear complex and fascicles. Journal of Neuro-Ophthalmology. 2000;**20**(2):138-144

[5] Simmons BD. Surgical management of ocular motor cranial nere palsyes. Seminars in Ophthalmology. 1999;**1999**:481-494

[6] Merino P, de Gomez LP, Villalobo JM, Franco G, de Gmez LR. Etiology and treatmen of pediatric sixth nerve palsy. Journal of AAPOS. 2010;**14**(6):502-505

[7] Dotan G, Rosenfeld E, Stolovitch C, Kesler A. The role of neuroimaging in the evaluation process of children with isolated sixth nerve palsy. Childs Nerve System. 2013;**29**(1):89-92

[8] Mahoney NR, Liu GT. Benign recurrent sixth (abducens) nerve palsy in children. Archives of Disease in Childhood. 2009;**94**(5):394-396

[9] Yuousuf SJ, Khan AO. Presenting features suggestive for later recurrence of idiopathic sixth nerve paresis in children. Journal of AAPOS. 2007;**11**(5):452-455

[10] Lyons CJ, Godoy F, ALQahtani E. Surgical management of sixth nerve palsy. Eye. 1987;**1**:78-85

[11] Price NC, Vickers S, Lee JP, Fells P. The diagnosis and surgical management of acquired bilateral superior oblique palsy. Eye. 1987;**1**:78-85

[12] Ehrt O, Boergen KP. A concept of the surgical treatment of trochlear palsy. Strabismus. 2004;**12**(2):75-83